Principles
of
Biochemical Toxicology

John A. Timbrell

Lecturer in Toxicology
School of Pharmacy
University of London

TAYLOR & FRANCIS LTD

London

First published 1982 by Taylor & Francis Ltd,
4 John Street, London WC1N 2ET.

Reprinted 1985

Typeset by The Lancashire Typesetting Co. Ltd,
Bolton, Lancashire BL2 1DB.
Printed and bound in the United Kingdom by
Taylor & Francis (Printers) Ltd, Rankine Road,
Basingstoke, Hampshire RG24 0PR.

British Library Cataloguing in Publication Data
Timbrell, John A.
    Principles of biochemical toxicology.
    1. Toxicology
    I. Title
    615.9   RA1211

ISBN 0-85066-221-4
ISBN 0-85066-319-9 (pbk.)

Contents

Contents

For Anna, Becky and Cathy

Preface

This book is intended as an introductory text for undergraduate and postgraduate students concerned with toxicology and allied subjects and for those involved in research and other areas of scientific endeavour who require a background to the subject of toxicology. Its primary purpose is to introduce the basic principles and mechanisms underlying the toxicity of foreign agents.

The idea for the book arose partly through the author's involvement with a course at the Royal Postgraduate Medical School, London, leading to the degree of Master of Science in Experimental Pathology (Toxicology). It became clear that there was no suitable text available for the toxicology section of this course, although there were a number of books which covered some of the areas of interest. Therefore, this book is primarily intended as a teaching text rather than as a research monograph. Consequently, it is not extensively referenced but has a bibliography of suggested reading in which more details of the topics and examples can be found.

The book is divided into chapters covering the underlying principles of the absorption, distribution, metabolism, excretion and dose–response relationships of foreign compounds. This is followed by chapters on the factors affecting the disposition of foreign compounds and the types of toxic effect they may cause. The final chapter is concerned with specific examples of toxicity in which the underlying mechanisms are generally understood, and these serve to illustrate the principles described in the foregoing chapters.

This arrangement should allow the student to progress through the book to achieve an understanding of the principles exemplified by the specific examples in the final chapter. Each chapter may also be consulted in isolation by readers requiring a basic account of a particular process, for instance drug metabolism.

A book this size is clearly not intended to give very detailed descriptions of the toxic effects and mechanisms of toxicity of more than a few carefully selected examples. It is hoped, however, that it will provide a useful guide and introduction to the rapidly expanding and increasingly important field of toxicology.

There are several larger texts available for more detailed information and references on certain aspects of toxicology and allied subjects. Particularly deserving of attention are *Casarett and Doull's Toxicology, The Basic Science of Poisons*, edited by Doull, Klaassen & Amdur (Macmillan, 1980) and *Principles of Drug Action*, by Goldstein, Aronow & Kalman (John Wiley, 1974).

I am grateful to Professor Robert Smith for persuading me to consider writing this book and for his critical review of the manuscript, and to colleagues and students who have knowingly and unknowingly contributed to its preparation. My thanks also to Sue Walker for typing the final draft so diligently.

Finally, special acknowledgement is reserved for my wife Cathy, who prepared virtually all the diagrams. Her patience in interpreting my hieroglyphics, diligence in typing, retyping and editing drafts, many helpful suggestions and above all encouragement, have made the book possible.

London 1981

Chapter 1

Introduction

Background

Toxicology is the subject concerned with the study of the noxious effects of chemical substances on living systems. It is a multi-disciplinary subject, as it embraces areas of pharmacology, biochemistry, chemistry, physiology and pathology, and although it has sometimes been considered as a subdivision of some of these other subjects, it is really a scientific discipline in itself.

Toxicology may be regarded as the science of poisons; in this context it has been studied and practised since antiquity, and a large body of knowledge has been amassed. The ancient Greeks used hemlock and various other poisons, and Dioscorides attempted a classification of poisons. However, the scientific foundations of toxicology were laid by Paracelsus (1493–1541) and this approach was continued by Orfila (1787–1853).

Development of toxicology as a separate science has been slow, however, particularly in comparison with subjects such as pharmacology and biochemistry, and toxicology has a very much more limited academic base, particularly in the UK. This may in part reflect the nature of the subject, which has evolved as a practical art, and also the fact that many practitioners have been mainly interested in descriptive studies for screening purposes or to satisfy legislation.

Scope

The importance of toxicology is growing rapidly with the increasing numbers of foreign chemicals, also known as xenobiotics, with which man is confronted. These include drugs, pesticides, environmental pollutants, industrial chemicals and food additives about which we need to know much, particularly concerning their safety. Of particular importance, therefore, is the ability to predict toxicity and this requires a sound mechanistic base to be successful. It is this mechanistic base that comes within the scope of biochemical toxicology, which forms the basis for all of the various branches of toxicology.

The development of toxicology has been hampered by the requirements of regulatory agencies which have encouraged the 'black box' approach of empiricism as discussed by Goldberg (see Bibliography). This routine gathering of data on toxicology, preferably of a negative nature, required by the various regulatory bodies of the industrial nations, has tended to constrain and regulate toxicology.

Furthermore, to paraphrase Zbinden, misuse of toxicological data and adverse regulatory action in this climate of opinion has discouraged innovative approaches to toxicological research and has become an obstacle to the application of basic concepts in toxicology.

Ideally, basic studies of a biochemical nature should be carried out if possible before, but at least simultaneously with, toxicity testing, and a bridge between the biochemical and morphological aspects of the toxicology of a compound should be built. It is apparent that there are many gaps in our knowledge concerning this connection between biochemical events and subsequent gross pathological changes. Without an understanding of these connections, which will require a much greater commitment to basic toxicological research, our ability to predict toxicity and assess risk from the measurement of various biological responses will remain inadequate.

Thus, any foreign compound which comes into contact with a biological system will cause certain perturbations in that system. These biological responses, such as the inhibition of enzymes, and interaction with receptors, macromolecules or organelles, may not be toxicologically relevant. This point is particularly important when assessing *in vitro* data, and involves the concept of a dose threshold, or the lack of such a threshold, in the 'one molecule, one hit' type of theory of toxicity.

Biochemical aspects of toxicology

Biochemical toxicology is concerned with the mechanisms underlying toxicity, particularly the events at the molecular level and the factors which determine and affect toxicity.

The interaction of a foreign compound with a biological system is twofold: there is the effect of the organism on the compound and the effect of the compound on the organism. It is very necessary to appreciate both for a mechanistic view of toxicology. The first of these includes the absorption, distribution, metabolism and excretion of xenobiotics, which are all factors of importance in the toxic process and which have a biochemical basis in many instances. The mode of action of toxic compounds in the interaction with cellular components, and at the molecular level with structural proteins and other macromolecules, enzymes and receptors, and the types of toxic response produced, are included in the second category of interaction. However, a biological system is a dynamic one and therefore a series of events may follow the initial response. For instance, a toxic compound may cause liver or kidney damage and thereby limit its own metabolism or excretion.

The anatomy and physiology of the organism affect all the types of inter-action given above, as may the site of exposure and entry of the foreign compound into the organism. Thus, the gut bacteria and conditions in the gastrointestinal tract convert the naturally occurring compound cycasin, methylazoxymethanol glycoside, into the potent carcinogen methylazoxy-methanol (figure 1.1). Administered by other routes, cycasin is not carcino-genic.

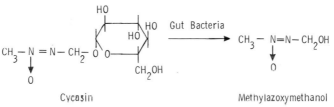

Figure 1.1. Bacterial hydrolysis of cycasin.

The distribution of a foreign compound and its rate of entry determine the concentration at a particular site and the number and types of cells exposed. The plasma concentration depends on many factors, not least of which is the metabolic activity of the particular organism. This metabolism may be a major factor in determining toxicity, as the compound may be more or less toxic than its metabolites.

The excretion of a foreign substance may also be a major factor in its toxicity and a determinant of the plasma and tissue levels. All of these considerations are modified by species differences and other genetic effects. The response of the organism to the toxic insult is influenced by similar factors. The route of administration of a foreign compound may determine the effect, whether systemic or local. For instance, tetraethyl lead causes a local effect on the skin if applied topically, but a systemic effect on the blood if it gains entry into the body. Only the tissues exposed to a toxic substance are normally affected, and consequently the distribution of a toxic compound may determine its target organ specificity, as does the susceptibility of the particular tissue and its constituent cells. Therefore, the effect of a foreign compound on a biological system depends on numerous factors, and an understanding and appreciation of them is a necessary part of toxicology.

The concept of toxicity is an important one: it involves a dàmaging, noxious or deleterious effect on a living system which may or may not be reversible. The toxic response may be a transient biochemical or pharmacological change or a permanent pathological lesion. The effect of a toxic substance on an organism may be immediate, as with a pharmacodynamic response such as a hypotensive effect, or delayed, as in the development of a tumour.

It has been said that there are no harmless substances, only harmless ways of using them, which underscores the concept of toxicity as a relative phenomenon. It depends on the dose and type of substance, the frequency of exposure and the organism in question. There is no absolute value for toxicity, although it is clear that botulinum toxin is very much more toxic than DDT on a weight-for-weight basis (table 1.1).

Table 1.1. Acute LD_{50} values for a variety of chemical agents.

Agent	Species	LD_{50} (mg/kg body weight)
Ethanol	Mouse	10 000
Sodium chloride	Mouse	4000
Ferrous sulphate	Rat	1500
Morphine sulphate	Rat	900
Phenobarbital, sodium	Rat	150
DDT	Rat	100
Picrotoxin	Rat	5
Strychnine sulphate	Rat	2
Nicotine	Rat	1
d-Tubocurarine	Rat	0·5
Hemicholinium-3	Rat	0·2
Tetrodotoxin	Rat	0·1
Dioxin (TCDD)	Guinea-pig	0·001
Botulinus toxin	Rat	0·00001

Data from Loomis, T. A. (1974) *Essentials of Toxicology* (Philadelphia: Lea & Febiger).

There are many different types of toxic compound producing the various types of toxicity detailed in Chapter 6. One compound may cause several toxic responses. For instance, vinyl chloride (figure 4.6) is carcinogenic after low doses with a long latent period for the appearance of tumours, but it is hepatotoxic after single large doses.

Investigation of the sites and modes of action of toxic agents and the factors affecting their toxicity as briefly summarized here is fundamental for an understanding of toxicity and also for its prediction and treatment.

For example, the elucidation of the mechanism of action of the war gas Lewisite (figure 1.2), which involves interaction with cellular sulphydryl groups, allowed the antidote, British Anti-lewisite or dimercaprol (figure 1.2) to be devised. Without the basic studies performed by Sir Rudolph Peters and his colleagues, an antidote would almost certainly not have been available for the victims of chemical warfare.

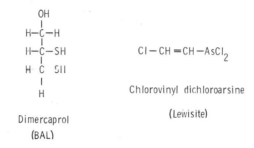

Figure 1.2. Structures of Lewisite and dimercaprol or British Anti-Lewisite.

Likewise, empirical studies with chemical carcinogens may have provided much interesting data but would have been unlikely to explain why such a diverse range of compounds cause cancer, until basic biochemical studies provided some of the answers.

Bibliography

ALBERT, A. (1979) *Selective Toxicity* (London: Chapman & Hall).

ARIENS, E. J., SIMONIS, A. M. & OFFERMEIER, J. (1976) *Introduction to General Toxicology* (New York: Academic Press).

CASARETT, L. J. & BRUCE, M. C. (1980) Origin and scope of toxicology. In *Casarett and Doull's Toxicology, The Basic Science of Poisons*, edited by J. Doull, C. D. Klaassen and M. O. Amdur (New York: Macmillan).

GOLDBERG, L. (1979) Toxicology; Has a new era dawned? *Pharmac. Rev.*, **30**, 351.

GOLDSTEIN, A., ARONOW, L. & KALMAN, S. M. (1974) *Principles of Drug Action: The Basis of Pharmacology* (New York: John Wiley).

HODGSON, E. & GUTHRIE, F. E. (1980) Biochemical toxicology; Definition and scope. In *Introduction to Biochemical Toxicology*, edited by E. Hodgson and F. E. Guthrie (New York: Elsevier-North Holland).

LOOMIS, T. A. (1974) *Essentials of Toxicology* (Philadelphia: Lea & Febiger).

PETERS, R. A. (1963) *Biochemical Lesions and Lethal Synthesis* (Oxford: Pergamon).

ZBINDEN, G. (1979) Application of basic concepts to research in toxicology. *Pharmac. Rev.*, **30,** 605.

ZBINDEN, G. (1980) Predictive value of pre-clinical drug safety evaluation. In *Clinical Pharmacology and Therapeutics, Proceedings of the First World Conference on Clinical Pharmacology and Therapeutics* (1980) (Macmillan).

Chapter 2

Dose–response relationships

Introduction

The relationship between the dose of a compound and its toxicity is central in toxicology. Paracelsus (1493–1541), who was the first to put toxicology on a scientific basis, clearly recognized this relationship. His well known statement 'All substances are poisons; there is none that is not a poison. The right dose differentiates a poison and a remedy', has immortalized the concept. Implicit in this statement is the premise that there is a dose of a compound which has no observable effect and another, higher dose, which causes the maximal response.

The dose–response relationship is a way of quantifying toxicity, and parameters gained from it may be useful for comparative purposes. It should be appreciated, however, that toxicity is a relative phenomenon and that the ways of measuring it are many and various.

Criteria of toxicity

The simplest measurement of toxicity is lethality, but this end-point is a relatively crude measure and gives little information about the underlying basis of the toxicity. However, it may be useful on a relative, comparative scale and it is important to know the limits of dosing for practical purposes. Consequently, a dose–response study using lethality as the toxic response is the starting point for most toxicity studies. The variability is usually considerable, as the end-point is often dependent on a number of physiological or biochemical processes. However, during such an initial study, observation of the animals may provide an indication of the toxic effect(s) produced by the compound, although it may or may not be the cause of death. It is therefore preferable to use a measure of toxicity which is as close as possible to the underlying mechanism. This may, of course, require prior knowledge of the target site, which may be a receptor, enzyme or other macromolecule, but an indication of the underlying cause of death or toxicity can sometimes be gained from an observation of the time-course of such effects after dosing. If an animal dies within minutes of the administration of a compound, it may well be that a major biochemical or physiological system has been affected.

The selection of a measurable index of toxicity in the absence of an obvious pathological lesion may be difficult, and the index may not relate to the overt toxicity or to the lethality. For instance, organophosphates may reduce blood cholinesterase, but this change may not be directly related to their toxicity. Similarly, the accumulation of triglycerides in the liver caused by hydrazine (figure 2.1) is not directly related to the lethality, this being due to another and probably unrelated effect involving the central nervous system. However, fatty liver induced by hydrazine is an example of a toxic response which can be readily quantitated and which shows a clear dose–response relationship. In this case, there is a graded, rather than an 'all-or-none' response, between a normal level of triglycerides in the liver and a maximum value. The fatty liver may be adequately assessed by measurement of the liver

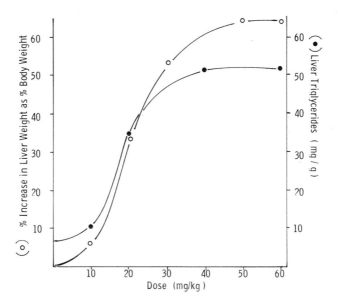

Figure 2.1. Increase in liver weight and liver triglycerides caused by hydrazine. Unpublished data of Scales & Timbrell.

weight (expressed as % body weight), a relatively simple measure which shows a similar dose–response relationship to triglyceride levels and which can be carried out at the same time as an initial toxicity study.

Conversely, the lung damage and oedema (water accumulation) due to the compound ipomeanol (figure 7.13), discussed in greater detail in Chapter 7, is directly related to the lethality. This can be seen from the dose–response curve (figure 7.15) and also when the time-course of death and lung oedema, measured as the wet weight : dry weight ratio, are compared (figure 7.14), strongly suggesting a causal relationship between them.

Clearly, some effects are reversible whereas others are irreversible. For instance, many pharmacological effects are reversible as are those toxic effects involving the inhibition of an enzyme, whereas direct tissue damage may be irreversible. These differences may be obvious during an initial investigation of toxicity, and may indicate likely mechanisms.

Dose–response

It is clear from the preceding discussion that the measurable end-point of toxicity may be a pharmacological, biochemical or a pathological change which shows percentage or proportional change or an 'all-or-none' type of effect such as death or loss of consciousness. In either case, however, the dose response relationship is graded between a dose at which no effect is measurable and one at which the maximal effect is demonstrated. The basic form of this relationship is shown in figure 2.2.

The dose–response relationship is predicated on certain assumptions, however:

(*a*) That the toxic response is a function of the concentration of the compound at the site of action;

(*b*) That the concentration at the site of action is related to the dose;

(*c*) That the response is causally related to the compound given.

Examination of these assumptions indicates that there are various factors which may affect the relationship.

Toxic response is a function of the concentration at the site of action

The site of action may be an enzyme, a pharmacological receptor, another type of macromolecule, or a cell organelle or structure. The interaction of the toxic compound at the site of action may be reversible or irreversible. The interaction is, however, assumed to initiate a proportional response.

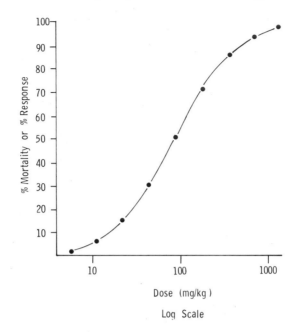

Figure 2.2. Dose–response curve.

If the interaction is reversible, it may be described as follows:

$$T + R \rightleftharpoons TR \ (\text{Response} \propto TR) \tag{2.1}$$

where T = toxic compound; R = receptor; TR = toxin–receptor complex.
When all the receptors are saturated, there will be the maximal response:

$$\frac{TR}{r} = 1 \ (100\% \text{ response}) \tag{2.2}$$

where r = number of receptors, TR = number of toxin–receptor complexes.

The number of receptor sites and the position of the equilibrium will clearly influence the dose–response, although the curve will always be of the familiar sigmoid type (figure 2.2). If the equilibrium lies far to the right (equation (2.1)), the initial part of the curve may be short and the slope steep. The intensity of the response may also depend on the number of receptors available. In some cases, a proportion of receptors may have to be occupied before a response occurs. However, when the interaction is irreversible, although the response may be proportional to the concentration at the site of action, other factors will also be important.

If the interaction is described as:

$$T + R \longrightarrow TR \tag{2.3}$$

$$TR \longrightarrow ?$$

the fate of the complex TR in equation (2.3) is clearly important. The repair or removal of the toxin–receptor complex TR may therefore be a determinant of the response and its duration.

From this discussion it is clear that the reversible and irreversible interactions may give rise to different types of response. With reversible interactions it is clear that at low concentrations occupancy of receptors may be negligible with no apparent response, and there may therefore be a threshold below which there is a 'no-effect level'. The response may also be very short, as it depends on the concentration at the site of action which may only be transient. Also, repeated or continuous low-dose exposure will have no measurable effect.

With irreversible interactions, however, a single interaction will theoretically be sufficient. Furthermore, continuous or repeated exposure allows a cumulative effect dependent on the turnover of the toxin–receptor complex. For instance, inhibition of cholinesterases by some organophosphates is effectively irreversible in some cases, and the half-life of the inhibited enzyme may be measured in weeks. Therefore, although an initial exposure might not give a detectable response, repeated exposure could lead to 50% inhibition, the level necessary for the toxic effect to be manifested.

With chemical carcinogens the interaction with DNA after a single exposure could be sufficient to initiate eventual tumour production with relatively few molecules of carcinogen involved, depending on the repair processes in the particular tissue. Consequently, chemical carcinogens may not show a measurable threshold, indicating that there may not be a 'no-effect level' as far as the concentration at the site of action is concerned. The existence of 'no-effect doses' for toxic compounds is a controversial point, but it is clear that the ability to measure the exposure sufficiently accurately and to detect the response reliably are major problems. Suffice it to say that certain carcinogens are carcinogenic after exposure to concentrations measured in parts per million, and the dose–response curves for some nitrosamines and for ionizing radiation appear to pass through zero when the linear portion is extrapolated. At present, therefore, in some cases 'no-effect levels' cannot be demonstrated for certain types of toxic effect.

With chemical carcinogens time is also an important factor, both for the appearance of the effect, which may be measured in years, and for the length of exposure. It appears that some carcinogens do not induce tumours after single exposures or after low doses but others do. In some cases, there seems to be a relationship between exposure and dose, that is, low doses require longer exposure times to induce tumours than high doses, which is as would be expected for irreversible reactions with nucleic acids. For a further discussion of this topic the reader is referred to the bibliography, particularly the articles by Weisburger & Williams (1980), Schmahl (1979), Zbinden (1979) and Lawley (Chapter 6).

Concentration at the site of action is related to the dose

Although the concentration in tissues is generally related to the dose of the foreign compound, there are various factors which affect this concentration. Thus, the absorption from the site of exposure, distribution in the tissues, metabolism and excretion all determine the concentration at the target site. However, the concentration of the compound may not be directly proportional to the dose, so the dose–response relationship may not be straightforward or marked thresholds may occur. For instance, if one or more of the processes mentioned is saturable or changed by dose, disproportionate changes in response may occur. For example, saturation of plasma-protein binding sites may lead to a marked increase in the plasma and tissue levels of the free compound in question. Similarly, saturation of the processes of metabolism and excretion, or accumulation of the compound, will have a disproportionate effect. This may occur with acute dose–response studies and also with chronic dosing, as for example with the drug chlorphentermine (figure 2.3), which accumulates in the adrenals but not in the liver after chronic dosing (figure 2.4). The result of this is accumulation of phospholipids, or phospolipidosis, in the tissues where accumulation of the drug occurs.

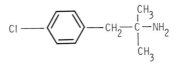

Figure 2.3. Structure of chlorphentermine.

The relationship between the dose and the concentration of a compound at its site of action is also a factor in the consideration of the magnitude of the response and 'no-effect level'.

The processes of distribution, metabolism and excretion may determine that none of the compound in question reaches the site of action after a low dose, or only does so transiently. For both irreversible and reversible interactions, but particularly for the latter, this may be the major factor determining the threshold and the magnitude and duration of the response. For example, the dose required for a barbiturate to induce sleep in an experimental animal and the length of time that that animal remains unconscious can be drastically altered by altering the activity of the enzymes responsible for metabolizing the drug. Similarly, changes in the plasma concentration caused by changes in the pH, and therefore the distribution of certain barbiturates, markedly alter the magnitude of the response. Both of these factors operate by altering the concentration at the site of action.

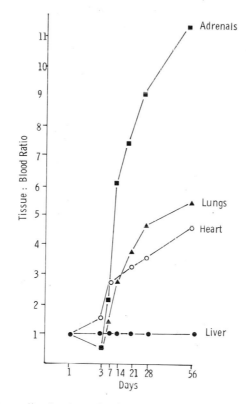

Figure 2.4. Tissue distribution of chlorphentermine on chronic dosing. Data from Lullman *et al.* (1975) *CRC Crit. Rev. Toxicol.*, **4**, 185.

Response is causally related to the compound

Although this may seem straightforward, in some cases the response is only indirectly related and is therefore not a useful parameter of toxicity to use in a dose–response study. This may apply to situations where enzyme inhibition is a basic parameter but where it may not relate to the overall toxic effect. Similarly, this criterion must be rigorously applied to epidemiological studies where a causal relationship may not be apparent or may not exist.

Measurement of dose–response relationships

Dose response curves may be derived by consideration of the population as a whole system or the consideration of the response in each individual.

The first type of treatment is obviously necessary where the end-point is an 'all-or-none' effect such as death. The second treatment may be applied to situations where there is a graded response to the toxic compound in the individual. Either treatment will give rise to the familiar dose–response curve (figure 2.2) when the percent response or percentage responding is plotted against dose. Thus, for the 'all-or-none' effect, the animals at each dose may be considered as parts of a single individual contributing towards the total percent response.

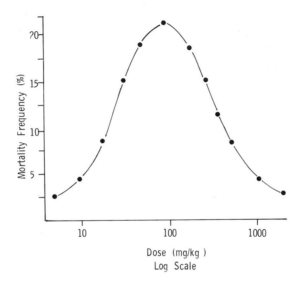

Figure 2.5. Dose–response relationship expressed as a frequency distribution.

The shape of the dose–response curve depends on a number of factors, but it is basically derived from the familiar Gaussian curve (figure 2.5), which describes a normal distribution in biological systems. This bell-shaped distribution curve results from biological variation; in this case it represents the fact that a few animals respond at low doses, and others at high doses, but the majority respond at around the median dose. The perfect Gaussian distribution gives rise to a symmetrical sigmoid dose–response curve. The more animals used, the closer the curve is to a true sigmoid shape. The portion of the dose–response curve between 16 % and 84 % is the most linear (linearity may be improved by using the $\log_{10}$ of the dose), and may be used to determine the parameter LD_{50}. The LD_{50} is that dose which is lethal to 50 % of the animals. However, for the conversion of the whole sigmoid dose–response curve into a linear relationship, probit analysis may be used, which depends upon the use of standard deviation units. The sigmoid dose–response curve may be divided into multiples of the standard deviation from the median dose, this being the point at which 50% of the animals being used respond. Within one standard deviation either side of the median, the curve is linear and includes 68% of the individuals; within two standard deviations fall 95·4% of the individuals.

Probit units define the median as probit five, and then each standard deviation unit is one probit unit above or below. The dose–response curve so produced is linear, when the logarithm of the dose is used (figure 2.6).

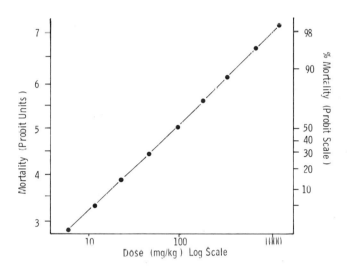

Figure 2.6. Dose–response relationship expressed in probit units.

The median dose or effective dose for 50% of the animals, or for a 50% response, may utilize pharmacological effect (ED_{50}), toxicity (TD_{50}) or lethality (LD_{50}). This value more accurately defines the dose than the TD_{95} or TD_5 (figure 2.7). The slope of the dose–response curve depends on many factors, such as the variability of measurement of the response and the variables contributing to the response. The greater the number of animals or individual measurements and the more precise the measurement of the effect, the more accurate is the TD_{50}.

The slope of the curve also reflects the type of response. Thus, a basic effect at the enzyme level gives a steep curve, if the effect itself is measured, or the effect is of general importance *in vivo*. For example, the toxic effect of cyanide involves the inhibition of the enzymes of the electron transport chain. This basic metabolic function is vital, and consequently gives a steep dose–response curve, reflecting a narrow dose range. Conversely, a less specific toxic effect with more inherent variables results in a shallower curve with a greater standard deviation around the TD_{50}.

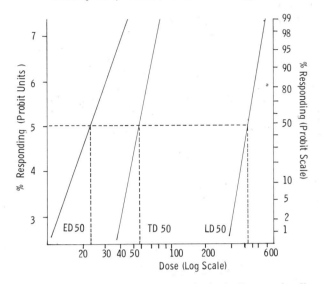

Figure 2.7. Dose–response curves for pharmacological effect, toxic effect and lethal effect, illustrating the ED_{50}, TD_{50} and LD_{50}. The proximity of the curves for efficacy and toxicity indicates the margin of safety for the compound and the likelihood of toxicity occurring in certain individuals after doses necessary for the desired effect.

The type of measurement made, and hence the type of data treatment, depends on the requirements of the test. Thus, measurement of the percent response at the basic level may be important mechanistically, with fewer variables, but for the assessment of toxicity, measurement of the population response may be more appropriate.

The value of the quantitation of the dose–response relation is mainly comparative. Thus, the therapeutic index may be a useful value. This index is defined as follows:

$$\text{Therapeutic Index (TI)} = \frac{TD_{50}}{ED_{50}} \text{ or } \frac{LD_{50}}{ED_{50}}$$

and relates the pharmacologically effective dose to the toxic dose, and hence indicates the margin of safety of a compound (figure 2.7). A more critical index is TD_1/ED_{99}. Similarly, comparison of two toxic compounds can be made using the TD_{50} (figure 2.8) and the dose–response curves, and this may also give information on possible mechanisms of toxicity. Thus, apart from the slope, which may be useful in a comparative sense, examination of ED_{50}, TD_{50} and LD_{50} may also provide useful information regarding mechanisms. Comparison of the LD_{50} or TD_{50} values of a compound after various modes of administration (table 2.1) may reveal differences in toxicity which might indicate what factors affect the toxicity of that particular compound. The dose of the compound to which the animal is exposed is usually expressed as mg/kg body weight, or sometimes mg/m² of surface

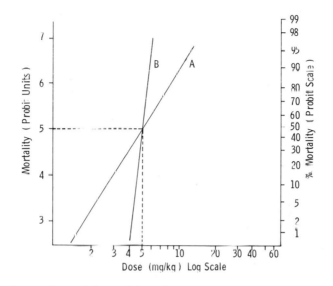

Figure 2.8. Comparison of the toxicity of two compounds, A and B. Although the LD$_{50}$ is the same (5 mg/kg), toxicity occurs with A at a much lower dose than with B, but the minimum to maximum effect is achieved with B over a very much narrower dose range.

area. However, because of the variability of the absorption and distribution of compounds, it is preferable to relate the response to the plasma concentration or concentration at the target site. This may be particularly important with drugs used clinically which have a narrow therapeutic index or which show wide variation in absorption.

It should be noted, however, that the LD$_{50}$ value is not an absolute biological constant as it depends on a large number of factors. Therefore, despite standardization of test species and conditions for measurement, the value for a particular compound may vary considerably between different determinations in different laboratories. Comparison of LD$_{50}$ values must therefore be undertaken with caution and regard for these limitations.

The value of the LD$_{50}$ test and the problems associated with it have recently been reviewed (see Bibliography, review article by Zbinden & Flury-Roversi).

Chronic toxicity

Chronic toxicity may be quantitated in a similar manner to acute toxicity, using the TD$_{50}$ or LD$_{50}$ concept. Measurement of chronic toxicity in comparison with acute-toxicity measurements may reveal that the compound

Principles of Biochemical Toxicology

Table 2.1. Effect of route of administration on the toxicity of various compounds.

Route of administration	Pentobarbital[1]		Isoniazid[1]		Procaine[1]		DFP[2]	
	LD_{50} (mg/kg)	Ratio to i.v.	LD_{50} (mg/kg)	Ratio to i.v.	LD_{50} (mg/kg)	Ratio to i.v.	LD_{50} (mg/kg)	Ratio to i.v.
Oral	280	3·5	142	0·9	500	11	4·0	11·7
Subcutaneous	130	1·6	160	1·0	800	18	1·0	2·9
Intramuscular	124	1·5	140	0·9	630	14	0·85	2·5
Intraperitoneal	130	1·6	132	0·9	230	5	1·0	2·9
Intravenous	80	1·0	153	1·0	45	1	0·34	1·0

[1] Mouse toxicity data.
[2] Rabbit toxicity data on di-isopropylfluorophosphate.
Data from Loomis, T. A. (1968) *Essentials of Toxicology* (Philadelphia: Lea & Febiger).

is accumulating *in vivo*, and may therefore give a rough approximation of the probable whole-body half-life of the compound.

For chronic toxicity, the TD_{50} or LD_{50} is measured for a specific period of time, such as 90 days of chronic dosing. The dose response is plotted as the percent response against the dose in (mg/kg)/day. If the TD_{50} values for acute and chronic toxicity are different it may indicate that accumulation is taking place. This may be quantitated as the chronicity factor, defined as LD_{50} 1 dose/LD_{50} 90 doses, where the LD_{50} 90 doses is expressed as (mg/kg)/day. If this value is 90, the compound in question is absolutely cumulative, if more than two, relatively cumulative, and if less than two, relatively non-cumulative.

The chronicity factor could of course utilize dosing periods other than 90 days.

An example of absolutely cumulative toxicity is afforded by tri-*o*-cresyl phosphate or TOCP (figure 2.9). This compound is a cholinesterase inhibitor and neurotoxin. In chickens, an acute dose of 30 mg/kg has a severe toxic effect, which is produced to the same extent by a dose of 1 (mg/kg)/d given for 30 days. This effect may of course be produced by accumulation of the compound *in vivo* to a threshold toxic level, or it may result from the accumulation of the effect, as it probably does in the case of TOCP.

Thus, the inhibition of cholinesterase enzymes by organophosphates may last for several days or weeks, and repeated dosing at shorter intervals than the half-life of regeneration of the enzyme leads to accumulation of the inhibition until the toxic threshold of around 50% is reached.

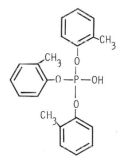

Figure 2.9. Structure of tri-*o*-cresyl phosphate (TOCP).

Bibliography

GOLDSTEIN, A., ARONOW, L. & KALMAN, S. M. (1974) *Principles of Drug Action: The Basis of Pharmacology*, Chapter 5. Drug Toxicity (New York: John Wiley).

HAYES, W. J. (1972) The 90 dose LD$_{50}$ and a chronicity factor as measures of toxicity. *Toxic. appl. Pharmac.*, **23**, 91.

KLAASSEN, C. D. & DOULL, J. (1980) Evaluation of safety: Toxicologic evaluation. In *Toxicology: The Basic Science of Poisons*, edited by J. Doull, C. D. Klaassen and M. O. Amdur (New York: Macmillan).

PAGET, G. E. (1970) *Methods in Toxicology* (Oxford: Blackwell).

SCHMAHL, D. (1979) Problems of dose–response studies in chemical carcinogenesis with special reference to *N*-nitroso compounds. *CRC Crit. Rev. Toxicol.*, **6**, 257.

WEISBURGER, J. H. & WILLIAMS, G. M. (1980) Chemical carcinogens. In *Toxicology: The Basic Science of Poisons*, edited by J. Doull, C. D. Klaassen and M. O. Amdur (New York: Macmillan).

ZBINDEN, G. (1979) The no-effect level, an old bone of contention in toxicology. *Archs Toxicol.*, **43**, 3.

ZBINDEN, G. & FLURY-ROVERSI, M. (1981) Significance of the LD$_{50}$ test for the toxicological evaluation of chemical substances. *Archs Toxicol.*, **47**, 77.

Chapter 3

Factors affecting toxic responses: disposition

Route of administration

It is clear that to exert a toxic effect a compound must come into contact with the biological system under consideration. It may exert a local effect at the site of administration on initial exposure, but it must penetrate the organism in order to have a systemic effect. The most common means of entry for toxic compounds are via the gastrointestinal tract and the lungs, although in certain circumstances absorption through the skin may be an important route.

Therapeutic agents may also enter the body after administration by other routes, and the following are the major routes of entry for foreign compounds:

(*a*) Skin;
(*b*) Gastrointestinal tract;
(*c*) Lungs;
(*d*) Intraperitoneal (i.p.);
(*e*) Intramuscular (i.m.);
(*f*) Subcutaneous (s.c.); and
(*g*) Intravenous (i.v.).

The site of entry of a foreign, toxic compound, with routes (*d*)–(*g*) being confined to therapeutic agents, may be important in the final toxic effect. Thus the acid conditions of the stomach may hydrolyse a foreign compound, or the gut bacteria may change the nature of the compound by metabolism and thereby affect the toxic effect. The site of entry may also be important to the final disposition of the compound. Thus absorption through the skin may be slow and will result in initial absorption into the peripheral circulation. Absorption from the lungs, in contrast, is generally rapid and exposes major organs very quickly. Compounds absorbed from the gastrointestinal tract

21

first pass through the liver, which may mean that extensive metabolism takes place. The toxicity of compounds after oral administration is therefore often less than after i.v. administration (table 2.1).

Transport across membranes

The major barrier to the absorption of foreign, toxic compounds is the cell membrane. This may be surrounding the cells of the skin, those lining the gastrointestinal tract or those of the alveoli in the lung. The passage of a compound across this membrane is therefore an important factor in absorption. The cell membrane, approximately 70 Å thick, is composed of proteins and lipids arranged in a bimolecular layer (figure 3.1). The protein may extend through the lipid and in some places pores may exist, which are basically polar areas containing water. There are a number of different ways in which foreign compounds may pass across cell membranes:

(*a*) Passive diffusion;
(*b*) Filtration;
(*c*) Facilitated diffusion;
(*d*) Active transport; and
(*e*) Pinocytosis.

The first mechanism, passive diffusion, is probably the most common for foreign compounds. It relies on diffusion through the lipid layer down a concentration gradient, and it does not show any substrate specificity.

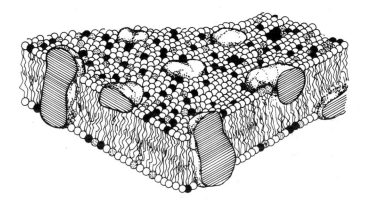

Figure 3.1. Schematic model of a biological membrane. Spheres represent the ionic and polar head groups of the phospholipid molecules, different types being represented as black, white or stippled. Zig-zag lines represent the fatty acid chains. Proteins associated with the membrane are represented by the large bodies with cross-hatching. Modified from Singer & Nicolson (1972) *Science*, **175**, 720.

In contrast, the filtration process relies on diffusion through the pores or aqueous channels in the membrane and is restricted to hydrophilic, low molecular weight compounds. Transport of foreign compounds through aqueous pores will depend on the flow of water through these channels and the sizes of the pores and the compound. This method of transport is usually restricted to small molecules. Pore sizes do vary, however, depending on the tissue. Thus, pores in the membranes of the kidney glomerulus may be as large as 40 Å in diameter, allowing large molecules to pass through, whereas most pores are 7 Å in diameter, restricting transport to molecules of around molecular weight 100.

Facilitated diffusion and active transport are both carrier-mediated, the former occurring down a concentration gradient, the latter against a gradient. Active transport therefore requires metabolic energy. Both processes may be saturated by the substrate and are specific for certain kinds of substrate, generally endogenous compounds, such as amino acids and sugars, or to foreign compounds which are similar to them. Thus, metabolite analogues such as fluorouracil (figure 3.2) may be transported actively.

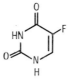

Figure 3.2. Structure of 5-fluorouracil.

Active transport systems may be saturated, the rate of transfer becoming zero-order and therefore independent of the concentration. Metabolic inhibitors block such transport and competition may exist between similar substrates. Polar molecules which would not undergo passive diffusion may be transported in this way, presumably by forming a complex with a specific carrier.

Pinocytosis involves invagination of the cell membrane around the foreign material. This may be an important process for the removal of large molecules or particles, for example from the alveoli in the lung.

Factors affecting transport

Passive diffusion of compounds through membranes depends on three basic factors:

(*a*) A concentration gradient across the membrane;
(*b*) The lipid solubility of the compound;
(*c*) The ionization of that compound.

Let us examine these factors in turn.

B

The concentration gradient

This is normally in the direction external to internal relative to the cell or organism. The rate of diffusion is proportional to the concentration gradient across the membrane, the area and thickness of the membrane and a diffusion constant which depends on the physicochemical characteristics of the compound in question. This relationship is known as Fick's Law. Passive diffusion is therefore a first-order rate process, being dependent on the concentration of the compound at the membrane surface.

Tissues with a large surface area and only a single cell membrane, such as the alveoli of the lungs, allow rapid passage of suitable foreign compounds.

It is apparent that an equilibrium will be reached when the concentration of the compound is equal on both sides of the membrane. In many cases, however, the system is a dynamic one, and the concentration on the inside of the membrane continuously changes as the compound passes into the bloodstream or other compartment or is changed metabolically or by ionization.

Lipid solubility

Passive diffusion relies on dissolution of the compound in the lipid component of the membrane and therefore only the lipid-soluble form of the molecule is transported. This is illustrated in table 3.1, which shows the

Table 3.1. Comparison between intestinal absorption and lipid : water partition of the non-ionized forms of organic acids and bases.

Drugs	Percentage absorbed	$K_{\text{chloroform}}$
Thiopental	67	100
Aniline	54	26·4
Acetanilide	43	7·6
Acetylsalicylic acid	21	2·0
Barbituric acid	5	0·008
Mannitol	< 2	< 0·002

Drugs were distributed between an organic solvent and an aqueous phase whose pH was such that the drug was largely in the non-ionized form.

Data from Hogben *et al.* (1958) *J. Pharmac. exp. Ther.*, **126**, 275.

lipid solubility of various compounds determined as the chloroform : aqueous solution partition coefficient and the degree of absorption through a bio-logical membrane, the intestinal wall.

The lipid solubility of a compound is an intrinsic property of the molecule. Solvents such as carbon tetrachloride, which are very lipid soluble, are rapidly and completely absorbed from most sites of application, whereas more polar compounds such as the sugar, mannitol (figure 3.3), are very poorly absorbed as a consequence of limited lipid solubility (table 3.1).

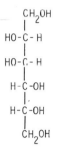

Figure 3.3. Structure of mannitol.

The degree of ionization

This determines the extent of absorption, as only the non-ionized form is lipid-soluble. The lipid solubility of this non-ionized form is also a major factor, as discussed above.

Thus, only the lipid-soluble, non-ionized form of a foreign compound is passively absorbed across a biological membrane. This is known as the pH partition theory.

The proportion of a compound present in the non-ionized form depends, in turn, on its pK_a and on the pH of the environment. (The pK_a of a compound is the pH at which 50% is ionized.) Therefore, knowing the pH of the environment at the absorption site, it is possible to calculate the amount of a compound which will be in the non-ionized form and therefore available for absorption.

According to the Henderson–Hasselbach equation, for an acid

$$pH = pK_a + \log \frac{A^-}{HA} \tag{3.1}$$

where $HA \rightleftharpoons H^+ + A^-$, and for a base

$$pH = pK_a + \log \frac{A}{HA^+} \tag{3.2}$$

where $A + H^+ \rightleftharpoons HA^+$.

As only HA in the case of an acid or A in the case of a base will be absorbed, the likelihood of a compound being extensively absorbed or not can be estimated from these equations, provided the pK_a and pH are known. For example, an acid with a pK_a of 4 can be calculated to be mainly non-ionized in acidic conditions, at pH 1. Rearranging the Henderson–Hasselbach equation (3.1),

$$pH - pK_a = \log \frac{A^-}{HA}, \text{ and}$$

$$\text{anti-log } pH - pK_a = \frac{A^-}{HA}$$

For an acid with a pK_a 4 in an environment of pH 1,

$$\text{anti-log } 1 - 4 = \frac{A^-}{HA}$$

$$\text{i.e. anti-log } -3 = \frac{A^-}{HA} = 0.001$$

that is $A^-/HA = 1/1000$ or the acid is 99.9% non-ionized.

Conversely for a base, pK_a 5 at pH 1,

$$pH - pK_a = \log \frac{A}{HA^+}$$

$$1 - 5 = \log \frac{A}{HA^+}$$

$$\text{anti-log } -4 = \frac{A}{HA^+} = 0.0001$$

that is, $A/HA^+ = 1/10\,000$ or the base is 99.9% ionized.

The same calculations may be applied to calculate the degree of ionization of acids and bases under alkaline conditions. It can easily be seen that weak acids will be mainly non-ionized and will therefore, if lipid-soluble, be absorbed from an acidic environment, whereas bases will not, being mainly ionized under acidic conditions. Conversely, under alkaline conditions, acids will be mainly ionized, whereas bases will be mainly non-ionized and will therefore be absorbed.

Because the situation *in vivo* is normally dynamic, continual removal of the non-ionized form of the compound from the inside of the membrane causes continued ionization rather than the attainment of an equilibrium:

$$H^+ + A^- \rightleftharpoons HA \overset{\text{membrane}}{\longrightarrow} || \longrightarrow HA \longrightarrow \text{removal}$$

If HA is continuously removed from the inside of the membrane, most of the compound will be absorbed from the site, provided its concentration at the site is not reduced by other factors.

Absorption

Skin

The skin represents an almost continuous barrier to foreign compounds; fortunately for the animal, it is not highly permeable. The outer non-vascularized layer consists of cells packed with keratin which limits the transport of compounds. The underlying dermis is more permeable and vascularized, but in order to reach the systemic circulation through the skin the toxic compound would have to traverse several layers of cells, in contrast to the situation in, for example, the gastrointestinal tract, where only two cells separate the compound from the bloodstream.

Compounds which are well absorbed percutaneously are generally very lipid-soluble, such as solvents like carbon tetrachloride which may exert a systemic toxicity following absorption by this route. Polar compounds, such as the small, water-soluble compound hydrazine, may also be absorbed through the skin sufficiently to cause a systemic toxic effect as well as a local reaction. The absorption of this compound may reflect its small molecular size (figure 5.19). Damage to the outer, horny layer of the epidermis increases absorption and a toxic compound might facilitate its own absorption in this way.

Lungs

Absorption via the lungs is an important route for toxic gases, volatile solvents, aerosols and in some cases airborne particles. The large surface area of the lungs is highly permeable to lipid-soluble and even some insoluble compounds. The blood flow is rapid and is separated by only 10 μm from the air in the alveolus. Consequently, volatile and lipid-soluble compounds are rapidly absorbed in solution by passive diffusion, and this depends on their lipid solubility.

Particulate matter, such as airborne particles of uranium dioxide, may be absorbed by pinocytosis.

The absorption of gases through the lungs is affected by the partial pressure of the gas in the expired air. The partial pressure of the compound in the arterial plasma water tends to approach that in the inspired air, and an equilibrium is achieved. The plasma water tension depends on the reaction of the gas with the plasma proteins, its ability to dissolve in lipids, and the distribution of the gas to other tissues.

Gastrointestinal tract

Absorption from the gastrointestinal tract is a major route of entry into the body for many toxic compounds and may occur along the whole length of the tract. The site of absorption for any particular compound depends on its physicochemical properties and the conditions in that area of the tract. The lining of the gastrointestinal tract essentially presents a continuous lipoidal barrier, passage through which is governed by the principles discussed above. Thus, in the acidic areas of the tract such as the stomach (pH 1–3), compounds which are lipid-soluble in the non-ionized form, such as weak acids, are absorbed, whereas in the more alkaline (pH 6) small intestine, weak bases are more likely to be absorbed. Using the Henderson–Hasselbach equation, the degree of ionization can be calculated and the site and likelihood of absorption may be indicated. In fact, both weak acids and weak bases are absorbed in the small intestine, which has a very large surface area.

Two important points to be considered with regard to absorption are as follows.

(*a*) The compound must be soluble in the non-ionized form. Thus, if it is a weak acid and largely non-ionized in the stomach, but is insoluble in the aqueous medium in the non-ionized form, it may be only slightly absorbed, despite its lipid solubility.

(*b*) Even though only a small proportion of the compound may be in the non-ionized form, as it exists in equilibrium, continual removal of that form by diffusion will continuously shift the equilibrium in its favour.

Let us consider the situation in the gastrointestinal tract, using benzoic acid and aniline as examples.

The pH of gastric juice is 1–3. The pK_a of benzoic acid, a weak acid, is 4. Taking the pH in the stomach as 2, and using the Henderson–Hasselbach equation as described above, it can be calculated that benzoic acid is almost completely non-ionized at this pH (figure 3.4):

$$\text{anti-log pH} - pK_a = \frac{A^-}{HA} = \text{anti-log } 2 - 4$$

$$\frac{A^-}{HA} = \frac{1}{100}$$

or 99 % non-ionized.

Benzoic acid should therefore be absorbed under these conditions and pass across the cell membranes into the plasma. Here, the pH is 7·4, which favours more ionization of benzoic acid.

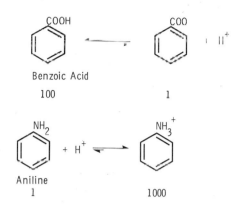

Figure 3.4. Ionization of benzoic acid and aniline at pH 2.

Using the same calculation, at pH 7·4:

$$\frac{A^-}{HA} = \frac{1000}{1}$$

or 99·9% ionized.

Therefore, the overall situation is as shown in figure 3.5.

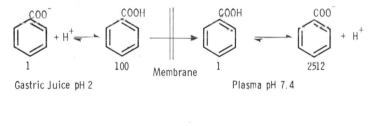

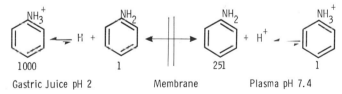

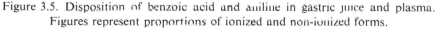

Figure 3.5. Disposition of benzoic acid and aniline in gastric juice and plasma. Figures represent proportions of ionized and non-ionized forms.

The non-ionized form of the benzoic acid crosses the membrane, but the continual removal by ionization in the plasma ensures that no equilibrium is reached. Therefore, the ionization in the plasma facilitates the absorption by removing the transported form.

Considering the situation for aniline in the same way (figure 3.6), for a base in the gastric juice of pH 2:

$$\text{anti-log } 2-5 = \frac{A}{HA^+} = 0\cdot001$$

$$\frac{A}{HA^+} = \frac{1}{1000}$$

or 99·9 % ionized.

Aniline is therefore not absorbed under these conditions (figure 3.5). Furthermore, the ionization in the plasma does not facilitate diffusion across the membrane, and with some bases secretion from the plasma back into the stomach may take place. The situation in the small intestine, where the pH is around 6, is the reverse, as shown in figure 3.6.

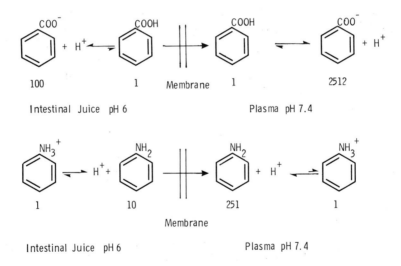

Figure 3.6. Disposition of benzoic acid and aniline in the small intestine and plasma. Figures represent proportions of ionized and non-ionized forms.

Therefore, it is clear that a weak base will be absorbed from the small intestine (figure 3.6) and, although the ionization in the plasma does not favour removal of the non-ionized form, other means of redistribution ensure removal from the plasma side of the membrane.

With the weak acid, however, it can be appreciated that although most is in the ionized form in the small intestine, ionization in the plasma facilitates removal of the transported form, maintaining the concentration gradient across the gastrointestinal membrane (figure 3.6). Consequently, weak acids are generally fairly well absorbed from the small intestine.

Strong acids and bases are not usually appreciably absorbed from the gastrointestinal tract by passive diffusion. The fact that some highly ionized compounds are absorbed from the gastrointestinal tract, such as the quaternary ammonium compounds, paraquat and pralidoxime (figure 3.7), indicates that specialized transport systems are probably involved.

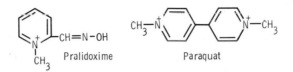

Pralidoxime   Paraquat

Figure 3.7. Structures of paraquat and pralidoxime.

Other foreign toxic substances known to be transported by specialized active-transport systems from the gastrointestinal tract are lead and 5-fluorouracil (figure 3.2).

Apart from influencing the absorption of foreign compounds, the environment of the gastrointestinal tract may also affect the compound itself, making it more or less toxic. For example, gut bacteria may enzymically alter the compound, and the pH of the tract may affect its chemical structure.

The naturally occurring carcinogen cycasin, which is a glycoside of methylazoxymethanol (figure 1.1) is hydrolysed by the gut bacteria after oral administration. The product of the hydrolysis is methylazoxymethanol, which is absorbed from the gut and which is the compound responsible for the carcinogenicity. Given by other routes, cycasin is not carcinogenic as it is not hydrolysed.

The gut bacteria may also reduce nitrates to nitrites, which may then react with secondary amines in the acidic environment of the gut, giving rise to carcinogenic nitrosamines and other compounds capable of causing methaemoglobinaemia.

Conversely, the acidic conditions of the gut may inactivate some toxins, such as snake-venom, which is hydrolysed by the acidic conditions.

Absorption from the gastrointestinal tract may be facilitated by the presence of food, particularly if it has a high fat content into which the compound may dissolve. In other cases, however, the presence of food may reduce absorption by retarding gastric emptying or by complexing with or sequestering the compound.

The absorption from the gastrointestinal tract is of particular importance, because compounds so absorbed are transported directly to the liver via the hepatic-portal vascular system. Extensive metabolism in the liver may therefore alter the structure of the compound, making it more or less toxic. Little of the parent compound may reach the systemic circulation in these circumstances. This 'first-pass' effect may be very important if hepatic metabolism can be saturated, and it may lead to markedly different toxicity after administration by different routes. Highly cytotoxic compounds given orally may consequently selectively damage the liver by exposing it to high concentrations, whereas other organs are not exposed to such high concentrations, as the compound is distributed throughout body tissues after leaving the liver.

Distribution

Following absorption by one of the various routes described, foreign compounds enter the bloodstream of either the systemic or portal circulation. Although only a small amount of a compound in the body may be in contact with the receptor or target site, it is the distribution of the bulk of the compound which governs the concentration and disposition of that critical proportion. The plasma concentration of the compound is therefore very important, because it often directly relates to the concentration at the site of action. Blood circulates through virtually all tissues and some equilibrium between blood and tissues is therefore expected. The distribution of foreign toxic compounds throughout the body is affected by the factors already discussed in connection with absorption. This distribution involves the passage of foreign compounds across cell membranes. The physicochemical characteristics of the compound and the particular tissue environment determine the distribution of the compound. The passive diffusion of foreign compounds across membranes is restricted to the non-ionized form, and the proportion of a compound in this form is determined by its pK_a and the pH of the particular tissue.

The passage of compounds out of the plasma through capillary membranes into the extravascular water occurs fairly readily, the major barrier being molecular size, and even charged molecules may therefore cross capillaries by passive diffusion. Therefore most small molecules, whether ionized or non-ionized, pass readily out of the plasma, either through pores in the capillary membranes or by dissolving in the lipid of the membrane.

Large molecules pass out very slowly, possibly by pinocytosis. The pores in the capillary membranes vary considerably in size, and therefore some capillaries are more permeable than others. Pore sizes of about 30 Å correspond to a molecular weight of 60 000. The exceptions to this are the capillaries of the brain, which are relatively impermeable. Passage across cell membranes from extravascular or interstitial water into cells is, however, much more restrictive.

Binding to plasma proteins

An important factor bearing upon the distribution of foreign compounds is their binding by the plasma proteins. Many foreign compounds are bound by these proteins, the most important of which is albumin. The binding is non-covalent, involving hydrogen, Van der Waals and ionic bonds, and the proportion of the compound bound depends on various physicochemical factors.

The non-bound (free) portion in the plasma is in equilibrium with the bound portion, but only the free compound passes through capillary membranes. Therefore, extensively protein-bound compounds (>90%) are restricted in terms of equilibration (distribution) within the organism. Under steady-state conditions, the concentration in the extravascular water equilibrates with the free concentration in the plasma.

Plasma-protein binding sites may be saturated, or one bound compound may be displaced by another. Thus, a dose threshold for toxicity may be seen as a result of saturation of plasma-protein binding sites. This results in a dramatic increase in the plasma concentration of the free compound. For instance, some sulphonamides become bound to plasma proteins, and in so doing may displace other compounds such as hypoglycaemic drugs like tolbutamide, giving an elevated plasma level of the free compound. The result of this displacement could be an exaggerated hypoglycaemic effect. Displacement of bilirubin by sulphonamides such as sulphisoxazole in premature infants may lead to toxic levels of bilirubin entering the brain.

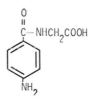

Figure 3.8. Structure of *p*-aminohippuric acid.

Although extensive plasma-protein binding affects passive diffusion, this being restricted to the free drug, it has little effect on active transport processes such as secretion at the kidney. For instance, *p*-aminohippuric acid (figure 3.8) is more than 90% bound to plasma proteins, yet it is cleared from the blood by a single pass through the kidney. This compound is actively secreted by the organic-acid transport system.

Thus, plasma-protein binding may affect distribution, prolong the half-life of the compound in the body, and be responsible for toxic dose thresholds.

Tissue localization

The passage of compounds into cells and across membranes is generally restricted to the non-ionized lipid-soluble form of the compound. Thus, foreign compounds which meet these criteria pass out of the blood, diffuse through tissues and are distributed through the body. Fat-soluble compounds may dissolve in tissues with a high fat content, and may remain sequestered there for some time.

For instance, the highly lipid-soluble anaesthetic drug thiopental (figure 3.9 and table 3.1) is rapidly taken up by body fat, and this distribution out of the tissues is one of the determinants of its short duration of action. The polybrominated biphenyls (figure 3.10) are industrial chemicals which accidently contaminated livestock and humans in Michigan in 1973. These highly lipid-soluble compounds are known to have become localized in the fat of the people and animals who were exposed.

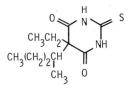

Figure 3.9. Structure of thiopental.

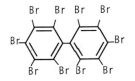

Figure 3.10. Structure of decabromobiphenyl.

Some compounds may accumulate in a specific tissue because of their affinity for a particular macromolecule, for example the binding of carbon monoxide to haemoglobin. These sites may be the target sites for toxicity. Accumulation may also occur in tissues other than the site of action, and tissues may sequester certain compounds with the help of endogenous compounds such as ligandin. This is a hepatic protein which binds carcinogens, steroids, bilirubin and a variety of exogenous organic anions, and which has been shown to be one of the forms of glutathione transferase.

Therefore, foreign compounds may be distributed throughout all the tissues of the body or they may be restricted to certain tissues. Two areas for special consideration are the foetus and the brain.

Passage of compounds across the placenta occurs generally by passive diffusion, and hence lipid-soluble compounds are readily transported. However, if metabolism *in utero* converts the compound into a more polar metabolite, accumulation may occur in the foetus. Foreign compounds generally achieve the same concentration in foetal plasma as in the maternal plasma water.

As mentioned earlier, passage across the capillaries into the brain takes place less readily than passage into other tissues. Ionized compounds will not penetrate the brain in appreciable quantities unless active transport systems are operative. Lipid-soluble compounds enter the brain with a facility dependent on their lipid : water partition ratio.

Plasma level

The plasma level of a foreign compound is an important parameter, as it relates more readily to the effect than the dose and is therefore a valuable piece of information to have in any toxicological study. In general, the plasma concentration more nearly reflects the concentration at the site of action, although the relationship may not be a simple one if the toxic compound is sequestered in a particular tissue or organ. For example, the drug chlorphentermine (figure 2.3) is found to accumulate in certain fatty tissues. This is because of its amphiphilic nature, which is the possession of both lipophilic and hydrophilic groups by the same molecule. Therefore, although the blood : tissue ratio is 1 : 1 for the liver after single and multiple doses, in the heart and lungs this is greater than one after one dose and reaches levels of around five after five doses (figure 2.4).

Volume of distribution

The animal body may be divided into various compartments: the plasma water, interstitial water and intracellular water.

The distribution of the compound into each of these compartments profoundly affects the plasma concentration. If a compound is only distributed in the plasma water (which is approximately three litres in man) the plasma concentration will obviously be much higher than if it distributed in all extracellular water (approximately 14 litres) or the total body water (approximately 40 litres) The volume of distribution (V_D) may be calculated from:

$$V_D = \frac{\text{dose (mg)}}{\text{plasma conc. (mg/l)}}$$

and is expressed in litres. A more rigorous determination of the volume of

distribution utilizes the area under the plasma concentration/time curve
(AUC) (figure 3.11) for the calculation:

$$V_D = \frac{\text{Dose}}{k \times \text{Area}}$$

where k is the elimination rate constant (see figure 3.13), or

$$V_D = \frac{\text{Dose}}{C_0}$$

where C_0 is the plasma concentration at time 0 gained by extrapolation of the
log plasma concentration versus time plot (see figure 3.13). Ideally, the compound should be administered intravenously, unless the degree of absorption
is known.

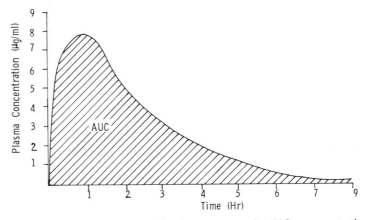

Figure 3.11. Plasma-level profile for a foreign compound. AUC represents the area
under the curve.

The volume of distribution is of course only a mathematical parameter,
but may yield useful information. For instance, a very high apparent V_D
may indicate sequestration in a particular tissue or localization in fat. The
total amount of a compound in the body, the total body burden, may be
estimated from a knowledge of the plasma concentration and V_D:

Total body burden (mg) = Plasma concentration (mg/l) × V_D (l)

The free rather than total amount in the plasma should be used for the
calculation of V_D, as only the former is available for distribution.

Distribution is a dynamic process, because the foreign compound is
absorbed over a period of time, and excreted at the same time. Obviously,
excretion depletes the plasma concentration, so there is a constant re-
equilibration between tissues and plasma.

Changes in the plasma pH may also affect the distribution, by altering the proportion of the compound in the non-ionized form, which will tend to cause a movement into or out of the tissues. (This may be used to treat barbiturate poisoning, for instance.) Phenobarbital, a weak acid (pK_a 7·2) shifts between the tissues (including the brain) and the plasma with changes in plasma pH (figure 3.12). Consequently, the depth of anaesthesia varies depending upon the amount of phenobarbital in the brain. Alkalosis, which increases plasma pH, causes plasma phenobarbital to become more ionized and upsets the equilibrium between tissues and plasma, causing phenobarbital to diffuse back into the plasma, as shown in figure 3.12. Acidosis causes the reverse shift. Administration of bicarbonate is therefore used to treat overdoses of phenobarbital. This will also cause alkaline diuresis and therefore increased excretion of phenobarbital into the urine.

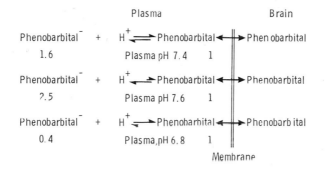

Figure 3.12. Disposition of phenobarbital in plasma at different pH values. Figures represent proportions of ionized and non-ionized forms.

Plasma half-life

The plasma half-life is also an important parameter which can be calculated from measurements of the plasma level at various time points. The half-life is the time taken for the plasma concentration of the compound to decrease by half from a given point. Measurement of the plasma level of a foreign compound at various times after dosing gives a curve which decays exponentially as shown in figure 3.11. Plotting this data semilogarithmically, as shown in figure 3.13, gives a linear relationship from which the half-life can be readily calculated:

$$\log C = \log C_0 - \frac{kt}{2\cdot303}, \quad \text{slope} = \frac{-k}{2\cdot303},$$

$$\text{half-life } (t_{\frac{1}{2}}) = \frac{0\cdot693}{k}$$

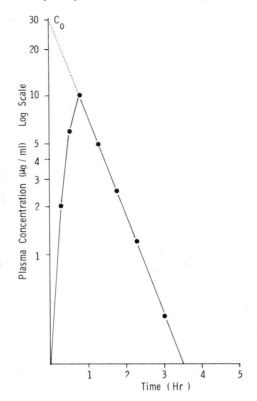

Figure 3.13. Semi-log plot of the plasma level of a foreign compound against time. C_0 is the plasma concentration at time 0.

where: C = plasma concentration; C_0 = plasma concentration at time 0; t = time after dosing; k = the elimination rate constant. A simple linear relationship is seen if the distribution of the compound fits a single compartment model. In some cases, however, a biexponential or two-phase decay is seen, as the compound first undergoes distribution and then the plasma concentration declines more slowly, governed by processes of elimination and metabolism. This may be described by a two-compartment model, or it may necessitate multicompartmental analysis. For a discussion of this topic, which is beyond the scope of this book, the reader is referred to the chapters in Goldstein *et al.* (1974) and by Tuey (1980) (see Bibliography).

The half-life of a compound reflects the various processes taking place *in vivo* following the administration of a compound. Thus, following the initial absorptive phase, the compound is distributed, metabolized and excreted, and these processes, acting in conjunction, determine the rate of removal of the compound from the plasma. Changes in the half-life of a compound may therefore give valuable information about changes in these processes. For instance, the half-life indicates the ability of the animal to metabolize and excrete the compound. When this ability is impaired, for example by saturation of enzymic or active transport processes, or if the liver or kidneys are damaged, the half-life may well be prolonged. For example, the minor analgesic paracetamol causes liver damage after large overdoses. After such excessive doses, the liver damage impairs metabolic capacity and consequently the plasma half-life is prolonged several-fold (see table 7.1). An indication of the ability of the animal to metabolize and eliminate the compound may be gained from the total body clearance. This may be calculated from the parameters described above:

$$\text{Total body clearance} = V_D \times k$$

or alternatively:

$$\text{Total body clearance} = \frac{\text{Dose}}{\text{AUC}}$$

where the dose is administered i.v. Examination of the plasma-level profile and kinetics of a compound after different routes of administration may yield valuable information, for instance indicating poor absorption or the occurrence of a 'first-pass effect'. For example, if the plasma-level profiles of a compound after intravenous and oral administration are as shown in figure 3.14, this may indicate either poor absorption from the gastrointestinal tract or a 'first-pass effect'. The 'first-pass effect' is the occurrence of extensive

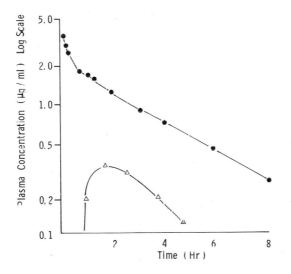

Figure 3.14. Effect of first-pass metabolism. Plasma concentration of a compound after oral (△) and intravenous (●) administration to the dog. Adapted from Smyth, R. D. & Hottendorf, G. H. (1980) *Toxicol. appl. Pharmac.*, **53**, 179.

metabolism during absorption and distribution from the site of administration. This most commonly occurs in the liver after oral administration, but may also occur in the gut wall during absorption and at other absorption sites. The extent of this first-pass metabolism may be as high as 70%, as in the case of the drug propranolol when given orally, and this means that the systemic circulation is only exposed to about 30% of the dose as the parent drug. A high apparent volume of distribution may be due to a 'first-pass effect'.

The plasma level and half-life are also important parameters if a compound is to be administered chronically. Thus if the dosing interval is shorter than the half-life, the compound accumulates, whereas if the half-life is very short compared with the dosing interval, the compound does not accumulate. The effects on the plasma concentration of the compound of these two situations are shown in figure 3.15.

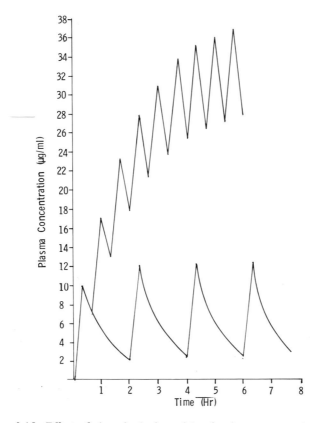

Figure 3.15. Effect of chronic dosing with a foreign compound on its plasma level. Half-life of compound is 1 h. Upper curve shows the effect of dosing every 30 min, lower curve the effect of a dosage interval of 2 h.

Ideally, for chronic dosing the dosing interval and half-life should be similar, so that a steady-state level is rapidly reached and the organism is exposed to a fairly constant level (figure 3.16). For steady-state conditions, the half-life determines the plasma level. That is, substrates with a long half-life attain a higher steady-state plasma level than compounds with shorter half-lives. It is obviously important to measure this plasma concentration for an assessment of chronic toxicity (figure 3.16).

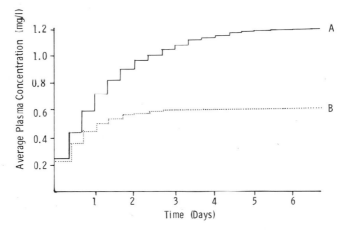

Figure 3.16. Average plasma concentrations of two foreign compounds after multiple dosing. Compound A, half-life 24 h; compound B, half-life 12 h; dosage interval in each case is 8 h. The accumulation plateau is directly proportional to the half-life, while the rate of accumulation is inversely proportional to the half-life. Adapted from van Rossum, J. M. (1968) *J. Pharm. Sci.*, **57**, 2162.

Excretion

The elimination of foreign, toxic compounds from the body is obviously a very important determinant of their biological effect. The more rapidly they are eliminated, the less likely they are to exert an effect. If, on the other hand, their retention in the body is prolonged, the potential for toxic effects is greater. The length of time a compound remains in an organism may be quantitated as the whole-body half-life, that is, the time required for half of the compound to be eliminated. This may be readily measured using the radiolabelled compound.

There are a number of routes of excretion, the major one being via the kidneys for most non-gaseous or non-volatile compounds. Other routes are via the bile, the lungs, and secretion into the gastrointestinal tract, or in fluids such as sweat, milk and semen.

Urinary excretion

The elimination of toxicants from the body via the kidneys into the urine is one of the most important routes of elimination. Toxic substances and other foreign compounds are removed from the blood as it passes through the kidneys, the blood flow representing 25% of the cardiac output. The processes responsible are passive glomerular filtration, passive diffusion and active tubular secretion. The physicochemical principles governing excretory processes are essentially as previously described for absorption.

The blood is filtered at the glomerulus and the filtrate passes into the tubules where reabsorption may take place for lipid-soluble, non-ionized compounds (figure 3.17). Filtration at the glomerulus normally occurs for most compounds of molecular weight less than 70 000, as the pores in the membrane are relatively large (40 Å). This filtration only applies to the non-protein-bound forms of foreign compounds. The concentration of the compound in the glomerular fitrate therefore approximates to that in the plasma in the unbound form. The state of the compound in the filtrate determines its subsequent fate. Thus, if the compound is non-ionized and very lipid-soluble, it passes through the membrane readily and is reabsorbed

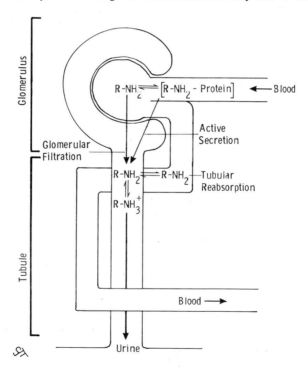

Figure 3.17. Schematic representation of the disposition of foreign compounds in the kidney.

into the bloodstream by passive diffusion. If the compound is ionized in the glomerular filtrate, or is polar, then it is excreted into the urine and the pH of the urine is obviously an important determinant of this. Therefore bases are more readily excreted if the urine is acid, and vice versa for the excretion of acids.

Passive diffusion of compounds through the tubules from the plasma into the urine is another mechanism of elimination.

In contrast, active secretion is an important mechanism of elimination for ionized compounds and is not markedly affected by plasma protein binding of the compound. This is because it is not concentration-dependent, unlike passive diffusion, and it is rapid; dissociation of the protein-bound compound continuously provides more compound for active transport (see page 33). Organic acids and bases appear to be transported by different secretory processes, which are located in the proximal convoluted tubules. The active secretion is an energy-requiring specific process which may therefore be inhibited by metabolic inhibitors or competitively by other organic acids or bases. Such competition may extend to endogenous compounds such as uric acid, and competitive inhibition of uric acid excretion may precipitate gout.

Factors affecting kidney function, such as age and disease, may obviously have a marked effect on the toxicity of compounds excreted into the urine.

Biliary excretion

Excretion of foreign compounds via the bile is a significant route of elimination for certain large, polar compounds. This route generally involves active secretion rather than passive diffusion, and there appear to be specific transport systems for organic acids, organic bases and neutral compounds. Quarternary ammonium compounds may be actively secreted into the bile by a separate process. This route of excretion seems to apply particularly to comparatively large, ionized molecules.

Such molecules are not readily reabsorbed from the lumen of the intestine or the bile duct itself if they are ionized at its prevailing pH. Compounds may therefore be effectively withheld from the systemic circulation if they are extensively excreted in the bile and are metabolized and conjugated rapidly in the first pass through the liver.

Large molecular weight conjugates are examples of compounds which undergo biliary excretion. The factors which influence biliary excretion are the molecular weight of the compound, its charge, and the species of animal in which the compound is being studied (tables 3.2 and 5.6). A molecular weight of greater than 300 is generally a prerequisite for biliary excretion, although this varies with the species concerned. The excretion of compounds via the bile into the intestine may lead to the reabsorption of the compound if the intestinal conditions permit. The most common mechanism for

Table 3.2. Effect of molecular weight on the route of excretion of biphenyls by the rat.

Compound	Molecular weight	Percent of total excretion	
		Urine	Faeces
Biphenyl	154	80	20
4-Monochlorobiphenyl	188	50	50
4,4′-Dichlorobiphenyl	223	34	66
2,4,5,2′,5′-Pentachlorobiphenyl	326	11	89
2,3,6,2′,3′,6′-Hexachlorobiphenyl	361	1	99

Data from Matthews, H. B. (1980) In *Introduction to Biochemical Toxicology* edited by E. Hodgson and F. E. Guthrie (New York: Elsevier-North Holland).

reabsorption is hydrolysis or metabolism of conjugates of the compound by intestinal microflora. This may result in the enterohepatic circulation of a compound (figure 3.18) or the reabsorption of another metabolite. This may, of course, have toxicological consequences, if the metabolite is more toxic than the excreted conjugate, or if it prolongs the half-life of the compound. It can be recognized by examination of the profile of the plasma concentration of the compound. The plasma concentration will not show a smooth decline, but will show increases after various intervals when reabsorption has taken place.

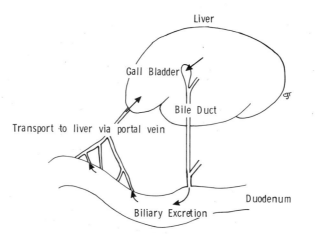

Figure 3.18. Enterohepatic circulation. The circulation of the compound is indicated by the arrows.

Some compounds are almost exclusively eliminated from the body by biliary excretion, and consequently toxicity may be markedly increased if bile secretion is impaired. One example of this is the toxicity of diethyl-stilboestrol. When this compound is given to rats with ligated bile ducts the toxicity, measured as the LD_{50}, is increased by a factor of 130, compared to non-bile-ligated, sham-operated, animals. As active transport is involved in biliary excretion, there is the possibility of saturation which may account for the occurrence of a toxic dose threshold. For example, the diuretic drug furosemide (figure 3.19) is hepatotoxic in mice at doses of around 400 mg/kg. This toxicity shows a marked dose threshold and it seems that it is partly due to saturation of biliary excretion and partly due to saturation of plasma-protein binding sites. The result is that the liver level of furosemide increases disproportionately with dosage, and the concentration of free drug increases from about 0·8 µg/ml at a dose of 80 mg/kg to 10 µg/ml at a dose of 400 mg/kg (figure 3.20).

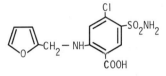

Figure 3.19. Structure of furosemide.

Lungs

Gases and volatile compounds are usually eliminated from the body by this route, as are the volatile metabolites of non-volatile compounds. The rate of elimination depends on the blood : gas solubility ratios, and takes place by simple diffusion, but generally it is fairly rapid.

Gastrointestinal tract

Passive diffusion into the lumen of the tract may occur for compounds which are non-ionized at plasma pH but which are ionized in the stomach, such as weak bases.

Milk, sweat and saliva

Milk, sweat and saliva are minor routes of excretion for some compounds. Because the pH of milk is 6·5, basic compounds may be concentrated in milk and this is of obvious importance in neonatal toxicity. Very lipid-soluble compounds, such as the polybrominated biphenyls (figure 3.10), may be extensively eliminated in milk.

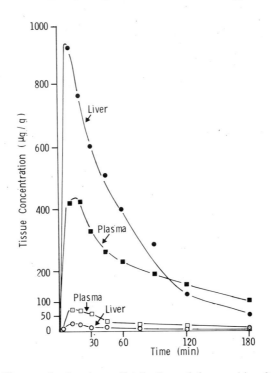

Figure 3.20.   Changes in the tissue distribution of furosemide after toxic and non-toxic doses were administered to mice. Closed symbols represent a toxic dose (400 mg/kg), open symbols a non-toxic dose (80 mg/kg). Squares are the plasma concentration, circles the liver concentration. Adapted from Mitchell *et al.* (1975). In *Handbook of Experimental Pharmacology,* Vol. 28, Part 3, Concepts of Biochemical Pharmacology, edited by J. R. Gillette and J. R. Mitchell (Berlin: Springer).

Bibliography

Absorption and distribution

ADAMSON, R. H. & DAVIES, D. S. (1973) Comparative aspects of absorption, distribution, metabolism and excretion of drugs. In *International Encyclopaedia of Pharmacology and Therapeutics,* Section 85 (Comparative Pharmacology), p. 851 (Oxford: Pergamon Press).

BRODIE, B. B., GILLETTE, J. R. & ACKERMAN, H. S. (editors) (1971) *Handbook of Experimental Pharmacology,* Vol. 28, Part 1, *Concepts in Biochemical Pharmacology* (Berlin: Springer Verlag).

CHASSEAUD, L. F. (1970) Processes of absorption, distribution and excretion. In *Foreign Compound Metabolism in Mammals*, Vol. 1, edited by D. E. Hathway, S. S. Brown, L. F. Chasseaud and D. H. Hutson (London: The Chemical Society).

GOLDSTEIN, A., ARONOW, L. & KALMAN, S. M. (1974) The absorption, distribution and elimination of drugs. *Principles of Drug Action: The Basis of Pharmacology* (New York: John Wiley).

GUTHRIE, F. E. (1980) Absorption and distribution. In *Introduction to Biochemical Toxicology*, edited by E. Hodgson and F. E. Guthrie (New York: Elsevier-North Holland).

JOLLOW, D. J. (1973) Mechanisms of drug absorption and drug solution. *Rev. Can. Biol.*, **32**, 7.

KLAASSEN, C. D. (1980) Absorption, distribution and excretion of toxicants. In *Casarett and Doull's Toxicology, The Basic Science of Poisons*, edited by J. Doull, C. D. Klaassen and M. O. Amdur (New York: Macmillan).

LA DU, B. N., MANDEL, H. G. & WAY, E. L. (editors) (1971) *Fundamentals of Drug Metabolism and Drug Disposition*, Chapters 1–7 (Baltimore: Williams & Wilkins).

SCHANKER, L. S. (1978) Drug absorption from the lung. *Biochem. Pharmac.*, **27**, 381.

SMYTH, R. D. & HOTTENDORF, G. H. (1980) Application of pharmacokinetics and biopharmaceutics in the design of toxicological studies. *Toxic. appl. Pharmac.*, **53**, 179.

Excretion

CAFRUNY, E. J. (1971) Renal excretion of drugs. In *Fundamentals of Drug Metabolism and Disposition*, edited by B. N. La Du, H. G. Mandel and E. L. Way (Baltimore: Williams & Wilkins).

MATTHEWS, H. B. (1980) Elimination of toxicants and their metabolites. In *Introduction to Biochemical Toxicology*, edited by E. Hodgson and F. E. Guthrie (New York: Elsevier-North Holland).

SMITH, R. L. (1973) *The Excretory Function of Bile* (London: Chapman & Hall).

Pharmacokinetics

GOLDSTEIN, A., ARONOW, L. & KALMAN, S. M. (1974) The time course of drug action. *Principles of Drug Action: The Basis of Pharmacology* (New York: John Wiley).

LEVY, G. & GIBALDI, M. (1975) Pharmacokinetics. In *Handbook of Experimental Pharmacology*, Vol. 28, Part 3, *Concepts in Biochemical Pharmacology*, edited by J. R. Gillette and J. R. Mitchell (Berlin: Springer Verlag).

TUEY, D. B. (1980) Toxicokinetics. In *Introduction to Biochemical Toxicology*, edited by E. Hodgson and F. E. Guthrie (New York: Elsevier-North Holland).

Chapter 4

Factors affecting toxic responses: metabolism

Introduction

The biotransformation of a foreign, toxic compound is an important aspect of its disposition *in vivo*. One of the results of such biotransformation is the facilitation of the removal of toxic compounds from the body, which, unless excreted, would accumulate to toxic levels. The types of biotransformations are many and varied and the metabolic systems involved are necessarily very flexible and non-specific. The major factor determining the route(s) of biotransformation is the structure of the compound itself.

As elimination from the body is the end-point for biotransformation, the metabolites so produced are generally more polar than the parent compound. Therefore, for excretion at the kidneys or for secretion into the bile, polar ionized compounds are preferred. Non-polar lipid-soluble compounds are reabsorbed from the kidney tubules or simply equilibrate between plasma and bile by passive diffusion, to no effect.

Biotransformation therefore often converts the parent compound into a more polar metabolite(s), which may be readily excreted. Consequently, the compound is eliminated from the body and accumulation to toxic levels is avoided.

However, if the chemical structure is changed from that of the parent compound, there will be consequential effects on the pharmacological and toxicological activity of that substance. The parent compound may or may not have pharmacological or toxicological activity, which may reside in the metabolite(s). Metabolism may therefore not necessarily be a detoxication process, in that the metabolites may be more toxic or active than the parent compound. The effects of metabolism are therefore often to facilitate elimination of the compound and alter its biological activity.

The effect of metabolism might just be to alter elimination from the urinary to biliary route, for example by increasing the molecular weight.

The metabolic alteration which takes place may not always increase polarity and water solubility. For example, sulphonamides are acetylated *in vivo* but the acetylated metabolites may be less soluble (table 4.1) and precipitate in the kidneys, causing toxicity. The pharmacological or toxicological activity of a foreign compound may be entirely due to a metabolite, as in the case of the antibacterial drug sulphanilamide, which is released from the parent compound prontosil by bacterial azo reduction in the gastrointestinal tract (figure 4.32).

Table 4.1. Solubility data for two sulphonamides and their acetylated metabolites.

Drug	Solubility in Urine (mg/ml at 37 °C)	Urinary pH
Sulphisomidine	254	5·0
	282	6·8
Acetylsulphisomidine	9	5·0
	10	7·5
Sulphisoxazole	150	5·5
	1200	6·5
Acetylsulphisoxazole	55	5·5
	450	6·5

Data from Weinstein (1970). In *The Pharmacological Basis of Therapeutics*, edited by L. S. Goodman and A. Gilman (New York: Macmillan).

Metabolism is therefore an important determinant of the activity of a compound, the duration of this activity and the half-life of the compound in the body.

Some very lipid-soluble compounds which are poorly metabolized may have whole-body half-lives measured in months or even years as is the case with the polychlorinated and polybrominated biphenyls.

The biotransformation of foreign compounds is catalysed by various enzymes, depending on the chemical structure of the compound in question. The most important is the cytochrome P-450 mono-oxygenase system, but numerous enzymes may be utilized, both those involved in intermediary metabolism and those whose main function is the metabolism of xenobiotics.

Although the major organ involved in the biotransformation of foreign compounds is the liver, other tissues and organs may be involved to a greater or lesser extent. The importance of the liver in this respect relates to its position as a portal to the tissues of the body. By metabolizing and hence removing toxic substances ingested orally and absorbed via the hepatic-portal circulation, the liver protects the organism. In some cases this metabolic conversion during the absorption phase is almost complete, resulting in a first-pass effect. The gut wall may also carry out biotransformation and hence be responsible for a first-pass effect, as may the lung for compounds absorbed by inhalation.

Types of metabolic change

Biotransformation may be conveniently divided into two types of reaction, phase 1 and phase 2 reactions. Phase 1 reactions are generally oxidative, reductive or hydrolytic processes which provide the necessary chemical structure for the phase 2 reactions, which are generally conjugations.

A foreign compound which possesses the necessary chemical structure for phase 2 reactions will be conjugated without undergoing a phase 1 transformation. For example, the lipophilic substance benzene undergoes phase 1 oxidative metabolism to phenol followed by phase 2 conjugation with sulphate (figure 4.1). If phenol is the administered foreign compound, it may immediately undergo phase 2 conjugation to yield the more water-soluble phenyl sulphate. It may also undergo further oxidative phase 1 type reactions.

Generally, therefore, the function of phase 1 reactions is to modify the structure of a xenobiotic so as to introduce a functional group suitable for conjugation with glucuronic acid, sulphate or some other highly-polar moiety, so making the entire molecule water-soluble.

Phase 1 reactions

The major phase 1 reactions are oxidation, reduction and hydrolysis.

Oxidation

The majority of oxidation reactions that foreign compounds undergo are catalysed by the microsomal mono-oxygenases, although mitochondrial and soluble fraction enzymes may also be involved.

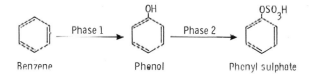

Figure 4.1. Metabolism of benzene to phenyl sulphate.

Microsomal oxidations may be subdivided into: aromatic hydroxylation; aliphatic hydroxylation; alicyclic hydroxylation; heterocyclic hydroxylation; *N*-, *S*- and *O*-dealkylation; *N*-oxidation; *N*-hydroxylation; *S*-oxidation; desulphuration; and deamination.

Non-microsomal oxidations may be subdivided into: amine oxidation; alcohol and aldehyde oxidation; dehalogenation; purine oxidation; and aromatization.

Microsomal oxidations

Oxidative biotransformations are a very important route of metabolism for foreign compounds. The majority of these oxidative reactions are catalysed by the microsomal mono-oxygenase system based on cytochrome P-450. This system, located in the smooth endoplasmic reticulum of cells of most mammalian tissues, is particularly abundant in the liver. Homogenization of liver tissue followed by differential ultracentrifugation separates the endoplasmic reticulum, and this microsomal fraction retains the cytochrome P-450.

The distribution within an organ may not be uniform however. For instance, in the liver the enzyme is most abundant in the centrilobular region (see Chapter 6) and in the lung the non-ciliated bronchiolar or Clara cells are thought to have relatively more of the enzyme than other lung cell types.

The mono-oxygenase system is based around the enzymes cytochrome P-450 and NADPH cytochrome P-450 reductase. Cytochrome P-450 is a haemoprotein and is the terminal oxidase involved in the hydroxylation of drugs and other foreign compounds and also of endogenous substrates such as steroids. There are a number of forms or isozymes of the enzyme, the relative proportions of which are determined by such factors as species and environmental influences. These isozymes are responsible for the oxidation of different substrates or for different types of oxidation of the same substrate.

At the active site of cytochrome P-450 is an iron atom (figure 4.2) which when in the oxidized form (Fe^{3+}) binds the substrate (S) (step 1, figure 4.2). Reduction of this enzyme–substrate complex then occurs, with an electron being transferred from NADPH via NADPH cytochrome P-450 reductase (step 2, figure 4.2). This reduced (Fe^{2+}) enzyme–substrate complex then binds

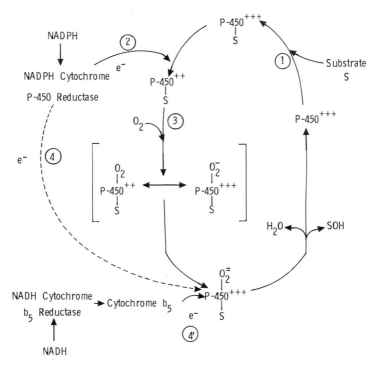

Figure 4.2. The cytochrome P-450 mono-oxygenase (mixed-function oxidase) system. P-450^{+++}: Cytochrome P-450 with haem iron in oxidized state (Fe^{+++}). P-450^{++}: cytochrome P-450 with iron in reduced state. S: substrate. e: electron. Adapted from Peterson & Holtzman (1980). In *Extrahepatic Metabolism of Drugs and other Foreign Compounds*, edited by T. E. Gram (Jamaica, New York: Spectrum Publications).

molecular oxygen in some fashion not yet entirely clear (step 3, figure 4.2), and is then reduced further by a second electron, possibly donated by NADH via cytochrome b5 and NADH cytochrome b5 reductase (step 4 or 4′, figure 4.2). The enzyme–substrate–oxygen complex splits into water, oxidized substrate and the oxidized form of the enzyme. The overall reaction is therefore:

$$SH + O_2 + NADPH + H^+ \longrightarrow SOH + H_2O + NADP^+$$

where S is the substrate.

Therefore, one atom of oxygen is reduced to water and the other is incorporated into the substrate. The requirements for this enzyme system are oxygen, NADPH and also magnesium ions.

Carbon monoxide, which binds with the reduced form of the cytochrome, inhibits oxidation and gives a complex with an absorption spectra peak at 450 nm, the origin of the name of the enzyme.

The state of oxidation of oxygen in the enzyme–drug–oxygen complex is at present unclear, but it may exist as hydroperoxide, O_2^{2-} or superoxide O_2^{-}.

Cytochrome P-450, although particularly important in the hepatic metabolism of foreign compounds, also has a role in the metabolism of endogenous compounds. Thus, the oxidation of certain fatty acids to their ω- and ω-1 hydroxy derivatives in the kidney and the hydroxylation of steroids in the adrenal cortex are two such examples.

Aromatic hydroxylation. Aromatic hydroxylation such as that depicted in figure 4.3 for the simplest aromatic system, benzene, is an extremely important biotransformation. The major products of aromatic hydroxylation are phenols, but catechols and quinols may also be formed, arising by further metabolism. Other metabolites such as diols and glutathione conjugates may also be produced. Consequently, a number of hydroxylated metabolites may be produced from the aromatic hydroxylation of a single compound (figures 4.4 and 4.5).

Aromatic hydroxylation generally proceeds via the formation of an epoxide intermediate. This is illustrated by the metabolism of naphthalene via the 1,2-oxide (epoxide) intermediate as shown in figure 4.5. The shift in the deuterium atom (^2H) that occurs during metabolism is the so called NIH shift. This indicates the formation of an epoxide intermediate, and is one

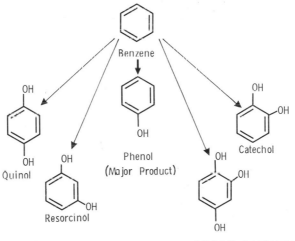

Figure 4.3. Aromatic products of the enzymatic oxidation of benzene. Phenol is the major metabolite.

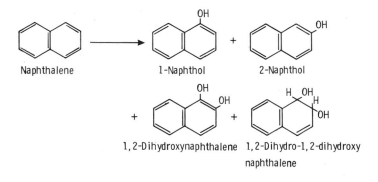

Figure 4.4. Hydroxylated products of naphthalene metabolism.

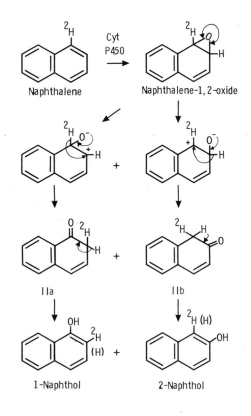

Figure 4.5. Metabolism of deuterium-labelled naphthalene via the 1,2-oxide (epoxide) intermediate, illustrating the NIH shift.

method of determining whether such an epoxide intermediate is involved. The phenolic products, 1- and 2-naphthols, retain various proportions of deuterium, however. The proposed mechanism involves the formation of an epoxide intermediate, which may break open chemically in two ways, leading to phenolic products (figure 4.5).

Each naphthol product may have deuterium or hydrogen in the adjacent position. The hydrogen and deuterium atoms (in 11a and 11b; figure 45) are equivalent, as the carbon atom is tetrahedral. Consequently, either hydrogen or deuterium may be lost, theoretically resulting in 50% retention of deuterium. However, in practice this may not be the case, as an isotope effect may occur. This effect results from the strength of the carbon–deuterium bond being greater than that of a carbon–hydrogen bond. Therefore, more energy is required to break the C-^{2}H bond than C-^{1}H bond, with a consequent effect on the rate-limiting chemical reactions involving bond breakage. Also, the direction of the opening of the epoxide ring is affected by the substituents, and the proportions of products therefore reflect this. The production of phenols occurs via a chemical rearrangement, and depends on the stability of the particular epoxide.

The further metabolism of suitably stable epoxides may occur, with the formation of dihydrodiols as discussed later. Dihydrodiols may also be further metabolized to catechols. Other products of aromatic hydroxylation via epoxidation are glutathione conjugates. These may be formed by enzymic or non-enzymic means or both, depending on the reactivity of the epoxide in question.

The products of epoxidation *in vivo* depend on the reactivity of the particular epoxide. Stabilized epoxides react with nucleophiles and undergo further enzymic reactions, whereas destabilized ones undergo spontaneous isomerization to phenols. Epoxides are generally reactive intermediates, however, and in a number of cases are known to be responsible for toxicity by reaction with cellular constituents.

With carcinogenic polycyclic hydrocarbons, dihydrodiols are further metabolized to epoxides as shown in figure 7.2. This epoxide-diol may then react with weak nucleophiles such as nucleic acids.

Unsaturated aliphatic compounds and heterocyclic compounds may also be metabolized via epoxide intermediates as shown in figures 4.6 and 5.17. In the case of the furan ipomeanol and vinyl chloride, the epoxide intermediate is thought to be responsible for the toxicity. Other examples of unsaturated aliphatic compounds which may be toxic and are metabolized via epoxides are diethylstilboestrol, allylisopropyl acetamide, which destroys cytochrome P-450, sedormid and secobarbital.

Aromatic hydroxylation may also take place by a mechanism other than epoxidation. Thus, the *m*-hydroxylation of chlorobenzene is thought to proceed via a direct insertion mechanism (figure 4.7).

The nature of the substituent in a substituted aromatic compound

c

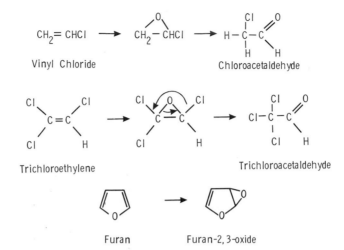

Figure 4.6. Metabolism of unsaturated aliphatic and heterocyclic compounds via epoxides.

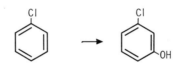

Chlorobenzene   m-Chlorophenol

Figure 4.7. *m*-Hydroxylation of chlorobenzene.

influences the position of hydroxylation. Thus, *o-p*-directing substituents, such as amino groups, result in *o*- and *p*-hydroxylated metabolites such as the *o*- and *p*-aminophenols from aniline (figure 4.8). Meta-directing substituents such as nitro groups lead to *m*- and *p*-hydroxylated products, for example nitrobenzene is hydroxylated to *m*- and *p*-nitrophenols (figure 4.8).

Aliphatic hydroxylation. Aliphatic hydrocarbon chains are not readily metabolized, except for those which are side-chains of aromatic structures. The initial products of microsomal enzyme-mediated hydroxylation are primary and secondary alcohols, as shown in figure 4.9. Thus, *n*-propyl-benzene may be hydroxylated in three positions, giving the primary alcohol 3-phenylpropan-1-ol, and two secondary alcohols. Further oxidation of the primary alcohol may take place to give the corresponding acid phenyl-propionic acid, which may be further metabolized to benzoic acid, probably by oxidation of the carbon β to the carboxylic acid.

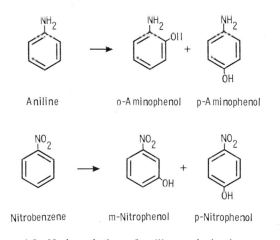

Figure 4.8. Hydroxylation of aniline and nitrobenzene.

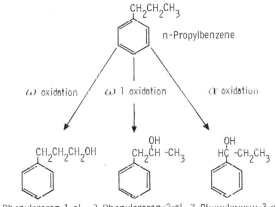

Figure 4.9. Aliphatic oxidation of n-propylbenzene.

Alicyclic hydroxylation. Hydroxylation of saturated rings yields mono-hydric and dihydric alcohols. For instance, cyclohexane is metabolized to cyclohexanol, which is further hydroxylated to cyclohexane-1,2-diol (figure 4.10). With mixed alicyclic/aromatic, saturated and unsaturated systems, alicyclic hydroxylation appears to predominate, as shown for the compound tetralin (figure 4.11).

Heterocyclic hydroxylation. Nitrogen heterocycles such as pyridine and quinoline (figure 4.12) undergo microsomal hydroxylation at the 3 position. In quinoline, the aromatic ring is also hydroxylated in positions *o-* and

C 2

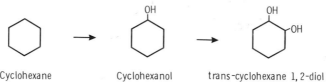

Cyclohexane   Cyclohexanol   trans-cyclohexane 1, 2-diol

Figure 4.10. Hydroxylation of cyclohexane.

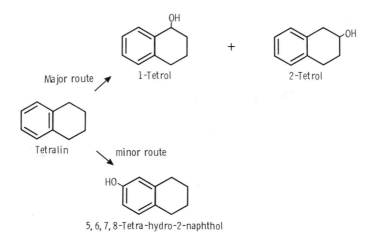

Major route   1-Tetrol   +   2-Tetrol

Tetralin   minor route

5, 6, 7, 8-Tetra-hydro-2-naphthol

Figure 4.11. Hydroxylation of tetralin.

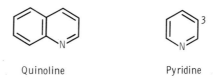

Quinoline   Pyridine

Figure 4.12. Structures of pyridine and quinoline.

p- to the nitrogen atom. Aldehyde oxidase, a soluble enzyme, may also be involved in the oxidation of quinoline to give 2-hydroxyquinoline (figure 4.13). Another example of heterocyclic oxidation is the microsomal oxidation of coumarin to 7-hydroxycoumarin (figure 4.14).

N-Dealkylation. Dealkylation is the removal of alkyl groups from nitrogen, sulphur and oxygen atoms, and is catalysed by the microsomal enzymes.

N-alkyl groups are removed oxidatively by conversion to the corresponding aldehyde as indicated in figure 4.15. The reaction may proceed via an unstable oxidized intermediate which spontaneously rearranges with loss of the

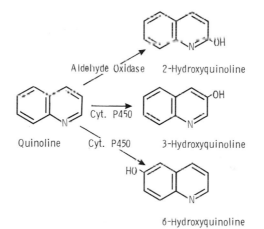

Aldehyde Oxidase   2-Hydroxyquinoline

Quinoline   Cyt. P450   3-Hydroxyquinoline

6-Hydroxyquinoline

Figure 4.13. Hydroxylation of quinoline.

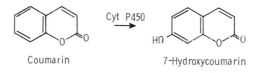

Coumarin   7-Hydroxycoumarin

Figure 4.14. Microsomal enzyme-mediated hydroxylation of coumarin.

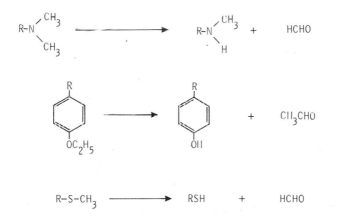

Figure 4.15. Microsomal enzyme-mediated *N*, *O* and *S* dealkylation.

corresponding aldehyde. The oxidative demethylation of *N,N*-dimethyl-aniline is illustrated (figure 4.16), two sequential reactions occurring in this case. *N*-Dealkylation is a commonly encountered metabolic reaction for foreign compounds which may have important toxicological consequences, as in the metabolism of the carcinogen dimethylnitrosamine (figure 7.3).

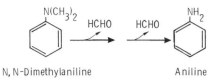

N, N-Dimethylaniline   Aniline

Figure 4.16. Oxidative *N*-demethylation of *N,N*-dimethylaniline.

S-Dealkylation. A microsomal enzyme system catalyses *S*-dealkylation with oxidative removal of the alkyl group to yield the corresponding aldehyde, as with *N*-dealkylation (figure 4.15). However, certain differences from the *N*-dealkylation reaction suggest that different enzymes may be involved. Figure 4.17 shows the *S*-demethylation of 6-methylthiopurine to 6-mercaptopurine.

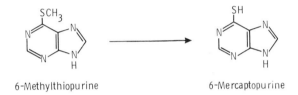

6-Methylthiopurine   6-Mercaptopurine

Figure 4.17. Oxidative *S*-demethylation of 6-methylthiopurine.

O-Dealkylation. Aromatic methyl and ethyl ethers may be metabolized to give the phenol and corresponding aldehyde (figure 4.15), as illustrated by the de-ethylation of phenacetin (figure 5.13). Ethers with longer alkyl chains are less readily *O*-dealkylated, the preferred route being ω-1-hydroxylation.

N-Oxidation. The oxidation of secondary and tertiary amines is catalysed by a liver microsomal amine oxidase which requires NADPH and molecular oxygen but which is not dependent on cytochrome P-450. For example, trimethylamine is metabolized to an *N*-oxide (figure 4.18). The *N*-oxide so formed may undergo enzyme-catalysed decomposition to a secondary amine and aldehyde. This *N* to *C* *trans* oxygenation is mediated by cytochrome

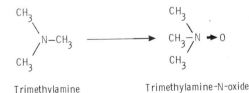

Trimethylamine   Trimethylamine-N-oxide

Figure 4.18. *N*-Oxidation of trimethylamine.

P-450, whereas the amine oxidase is a mixed-function oxidase involving a flavoprotein which is not NADPH cytochrome P 450 reductase.

N,N dimethylaniline would also be a substrate for this amine oxidase as well as for microsomal dealkylation (figure 4.16).

N-Hydroxylation. N-hydroxylation of primary arylamines, arylamides and hydrazines is also catalysed by a microsomal mixed-function oxidase involving cytochrome P-450 and requiring NADPH and molecular oxygen. Thus, the N-hydroxylation of aniline is as shown in figure 4.19. The N-hydroxylated product, phenylhydroxylamine, is thought to be responsible for the production of methaemoglobinaemia after aniline administration to experimental animals. This may occur by further oxidation of phenylhydroxylamine to nitrosobenzene which may then be reduced back to phenylhydroxylamine. This reaction lowers the reduced glutathione concentration in the red blood cell, removing the protection of haemoglobin against oxidative damage.

N-hydroxylated products may be chemically unstable and dehydrate, as does phenylhydroxylamine, thereby producing a reactive electrophile such as an imine or imino-quinone (figure 7.8).

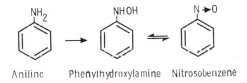

Aniline   Phenylhydroxylamine   Nitrosobenzene

Figure 4.19. *N*-Hydroxylation of aniline.

An important example toxicologically is the *N*-hydroxylation of 2-acetylaminofluorene (figure 4.20). N-hydroxylation is one of the reactions responsible for converting the compound into a potent carcinogen. A second example is the N-hydroxylation of isopropylhydrazine, thought to be involved in the production of a hepatotoxic intermediate (figure 7.12).

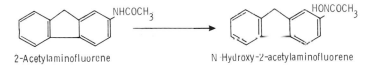

2-Acetylaminofluorene   N-Hydroxy-2-acetylaminofluorene

Figure 4.20. *N*-Hydroxylation of 2-acetylaminofluorene.

S-Oxidation. Aromatic and aliphatic sulphides or thioethers may undergo oxidation to form sulphoxides and then, after further oxidation, sulphones (figure 4.21). This is catalysed by a microsomal mono-oxygenase requiring

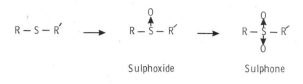

Sulphoxide   Sulphone

Figure 4.21. *S*-Oxidation to form a sulphoxide and sulphone.

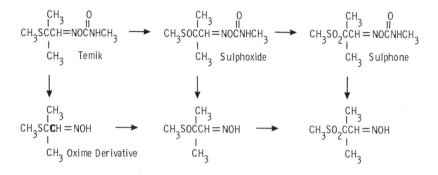

Figure 4.22. Metabolism of the pesticide temik.

NADPH and cytochrome P-450. A number of foreign compounds, for example drugs like chlorpromazine and various pesticides such as temik (figure 4.22), undergo this reaction.

Desulphuration. Replacement of sulphur by oxygen is known to occur in a number of cases, and the oxygenation of the insecticide parathion to give the more toxic paraoxon is a good example of this (figure 4.23). This reaction is also important for other phosphorothionate insecticides. The toxicity depends upon inhibition of cholinesterases and the oxidized product is much more potent in this respect. The reaction appears to involve a microsomal mono-oxygenase, dependent on NADPH and oxygen.

Oxidative desulphuration at the C–S bond may also occur, such as in the barbiturate thiopental, which is metabolized to pentobarbital, or in the metabolism of phenylthiourea to phenylurea (figure 4.24).

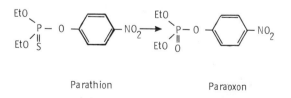

Parathion   Paraoxon

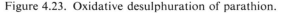

Figure 4.23. Oxidative desulphuration of parathion.

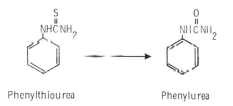

Phenylthiourea   Phenylurea

Figure 4.24. Oxidative desulphuration of phenylthiourea.

Deamination. Deamination of a compound such as amphetamine may be catalysed by a microsomal amine oxidase which requires NADPH and molecular oxygen. The product of deamination of a primary amine is the corresponding ketone (figure 4.25). This overall reaction may in fact represent several steps; initial carbon oxidation followed by rearrangement to give the ketone with the loss of ammonia. Therefore, the metabolic reaction is carbon oxidation rather than oxidation at the nitrogen atom.

(Monoamine oxidase, which may also be involved in the deamination of amines, is a mitochondrial enzyme.)

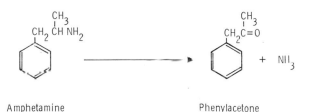

Amphetamine   Phenylacetone

Figure 4.25. Oxidative deamination of amphetamine.

Non-microsomal oxidation

Amine oxidation. Monoamine oxidase and diamine oxidase are both involved in the oxidative deamination of primary, secondary and tertiary amines such as the endogenous compounds 5-hydroxytryptamine and diamines such as putrescine (figure 4.26). The products of oxidation of both monoamines and diamines are aldehydes.

The monoamine oxidase enzyme is located in the mitochondria of a number of tissues and diamine oxidase is a soluble enzyme also found in a number of tissues.

Secondary and tertiary amines are less readily deaminated, being preferentially dealkylated to primary amines.

Alcohol and aldehyde oxidation. Although *in vitro* a microsomal enzyme system has been demonstrated which oxidizes ethanol, probably the more

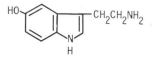

5-Hydroxytryptamine

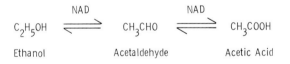

Putrescine

Figure 4.26. Structure of 5-hydroxytryptamine and putrescine, substrates for monoamine and diamine oxidase respectively.

important enzyme *in vivo* is alcohol dehydrogenase, which is found in the soluble fraction in various tissues. The coenzyme for this fairly non-specific enzyme is usually NAD, although NADP may also be utilized.

The product of the oxidation is the corresponding aldehyde if the substrate is a primary alcohol (figure 4.27) or a ketone if a secondary alcohol is oxidized. Secondary alcohols are oxidized much more slowly than primary alcohols, however. The aldehyde produced by this oxidation may be further oxidized by aldehyde dehydrogenase to the corresponding acid. This enzyme also requires NAD and is found in the soluble fraction. Alcohol dehydrogenase may have a role in the hepatotoxicity of allyl alcohol. This alcohol causes periportal necrosis (see page 132) in experimental animals; this is thought to be due to metabolism to allyl aldehyde (acrolein) (figure 4.28).

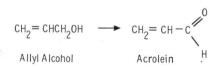

Figure 4.27. Oxidation of ethanol by alcohol dehydrogenase.

$$CH_2 = CHCH_2OH \longrightarrow CH_2 = CH - C \overset{\displaystyle O}{\underset{\displaystyle H}{\diagdown}}$$

Allyl Alcohol   Acrolein

Figure 4.28. Alcohol dehydrogenase-catalysed oxidation of allyl alcohol.

Other enzymes may also be involved in the oxidation of aldehydes, particularly aldehyde oxidase and xanthine oxidase. These enzymes are both found in the soluble fraction of the cell, contain molybdenum and utilize flavoproteins. Xanthine oxidase is also involved in the oxidation of purines.

Purine oxidation. The oxidation of purines and purine derivatives is probably catalysed by xanthine oxidase. For example, the enzyme oxidizes hypoxanthine to xanthine and thence uric acid (figure 4.29). Xanthine oxidase also catalyses the oxidation of foreign compounds, such as the nitrogen heterocycle phthalazine (figure 4.30). This compound is also a substrate for aldehyde oxidase, giving the same product.

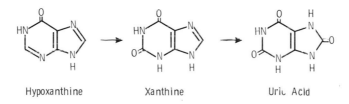

Hypoxanthine   Xanthine   Uric Acid

Figure 4.29. Oxidation of hypoxanthine by xanthine oxidase.

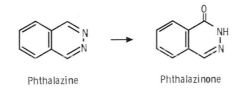

Phthalazine   Phthalazinone

Figure 4.30. Oxidation of phthalazine by xanthine oxidase.

Aromatization of alicyclic compounds. Cyclohexane carboxylic acids may be metabolized by a mitochondrial enzyme system to an aromatic acid such as benzoic acid. This enzyme system requires CoA, ATP and oxygen and is thought to involve three sequential dehydrogenation steps after the initial formation of the cyclohexanoyl CoA (figure 4.31).

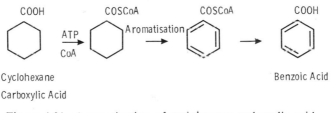

Cyclohexane
Carboxylic Acid   Benzoic Acid

Figure 4.31 Aromatization of cyclohexane carboxylic acid

Reduction

The enzymes responsible for reduction may be located in both the microsomal fraction and the soluble cell fraction. The location of the reductase depends on the particular type of reduction being catalysed.

There are probably a number of reductases which catalyse the reduction of azo and nitro compounds. Some of these reductases are microsomal enzymes and involve the coenzyme FAD, whereas others are found in the soluble fraction. The reductions catalysed take place under anaerobic conditions and are dependent upon NADH or NADPH. The involvement of FAD may simply be as a non-enzymic electron donor.

The reduction of the azo dye prontosil is a well known example of azo reduction. This reaction is carried out by the reductases in the gut bacteria and produces the antibacterial drug sulphanilamide (figure 4.32). The gut microflora may play an important part in the reduction of many azo compounds.

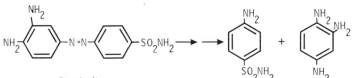

Prontosil

Sulphanilamide

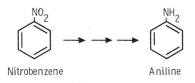

Nitrobenzene   Aniline

Figure 4.32. Reduction of the azo group in prontosil and the nitro group in nitrobenzene.

The reduction of nitro compounds proceeds through several stages to yield the fully reduced primary amine, as illustrated with nitrobenzene (figure 4.32). The intermediates are nitrosobenzene and phenylhydroxylamine. Aryl-hydroxylamines, whether derived from nitro compounds by reduction or by *N*-hydroxylation of amines, have been shown to play a very important role in the toxicity of a number of compounds. An important example is the reduction of nitroquinoline *N*-oxide. This proceeds via the hydroxylamine, which is an extremely carcinogenic metabolite, probably the ultimate carcinogen (figure 4.33).

Other reductive biotransformations not catalysed by microsomal enzymes are known. These include the reduction of aldehydes and ketones, the reduction of double bonds, and the reduction of *S*- and *N*-oxides, *N*-hydroxy compounds and disulphides.

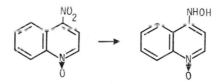

Nitroquinoline-N-oxide   Hydroxylaminoquinoline-N-oxide

Figure 4.33. Reduction of nitroquinoline-*N*-oxide.

Dehalogenation

The microsomal enzyme-mediated removal of a halogen atom from a foreign compound may be either oxidative or reductive. For example, the volatile anaesthetic halothane undergoes both oxidative and reductive dehalogenation (figures 4.34 and 4.35). The latter metabolic pathway is possibly responsible for the occasional hepatoxicity of the drug. It seems that there are several metabolic pathways, some occurring under anaerobic conditions, others under aerobic conditions.

Carbon tetrachloride also undergoes reductive dechlorination to give chloroform (figure 7.4). This is catalysed by the cytochrome P-450 system *in vitro* under anaerobic conditions and probably involves a free-radical reaction (see Chapter 7).

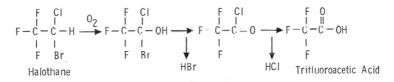

Figure 4.34. Oxidative metabolism of halothane.

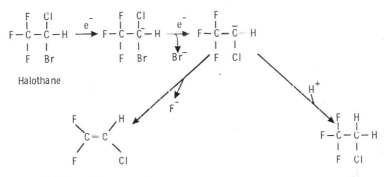

Figure 4.35. Reductive metabolism of halothane.

Dehalogenation may also involve glutathione, as in the dehydrohalogenation of the insecticide DDT (figure 4.36).

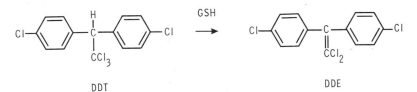

DDT   DDE

Figure 4.36. Dehydrohalogenation of DDT.

Hydrolysis

Esters and amides are generally metabolized by hydrolysis. The enzymes which catalyse these hydrolytic reactions, esterases and amidases, are found in a variety of tissues, including the plasma, usually in the soluble fraction of the cell. There are numerous hydrolytic enzymes with different substrate specificities.

Hydrolysis of esters

Various esterases exist in mammalian tissues, hydrolysing different types of esters. These enzymes are classified as aryl esterases (aromatic esters), alkyl esterases (aliphatic esters), choline esterases and acetyl esterases. Other enzymes such as trypsin and chymotrypsin may also hydrolyse certain carboxyl esters (figure 4.37).

$$RCOOR' \ + \ H_2O \ \longrightarrow \ RCOOH \ + \ R'OH$$

Figure 4.37. Ester hydrolysis.

Metabolism of the local anaesthetic procaine provides an example of esterase action, as shown in figure 4.38. This hydrolysis may be carried out by both a plasma esterase and a microsomal enzyme. The insecticide malathion is metabolized by a carboxyl esterase in mammals, rather than undergoing oxidative desulphuration as in insects (figure 5.7).

Hydrolysis of amides

The amidase-catalysed hydrolysis of amides is rather slower than that of esters. Thus, unlike procaine, the analogue procainamide is not hydrolysed

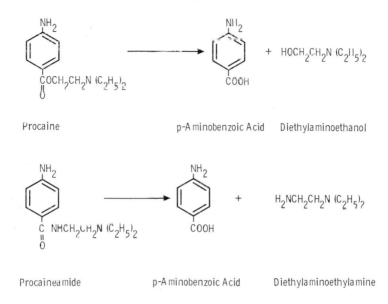

Procaine   p-Aminobenzoic Acid   Diethylaminoethanol

Procaineamide   p-Aminobenzoic Acid   Diethylaminoethylamine

Figure 4.38. Hydrolysis of the ester procaine and the amide procainamide.

in the plasma at all, the hydrolysis *in vivo* being carried out by enzymes in other tissues (figure 4.38).

The hydrolysis of some amides may be catalysed by a liver microsomal carboxyl esterase, as is the case with phenacetin (figure 4.39). Hydrolysis of the acetylamino group resulting in deacetylation is known to be important in the toxicity of a number of compounds. For example, the deacetylated metabolites of phenacetin are thought to be responsible for its toxicity, the oxidation of haemoglobin to methaemoglobin. This toxic effect occasionally occurs in subjects taking therapeutic doses of the drug who have a deficiency in the normal pathway of metabolism of phenacetin to paracetamol. Consequently, more phenacetin is metabolized by deacetylation and subsequent oxidation to toxic metabolites (figure 5.13).

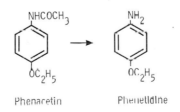

Phenacetin   Phenetidine

Figure 4.39. Deacetylation of phenacetin.

Hydrolysis of hydrazides

The drug isoniazid (isonicotinic acid hydrazide) is hydrolysed *in vivo* to the corresponding acid and hydrazine, as shown in figure 4.40. However, in man, *in vivo*, hydrolysis of the acetylated metabolite acetylisoniazid is quantitatively more important and toxicologically more significant (figure 4.41). This hydrolysis reaction accounts for about 45% of the acetylisoniazid produced. These hydrolysis reactions are probably catalysed by amidases and are inhibited by organophosphate inhibitors such as bis-*p*-nitrophenyl phosphate (figure 5.21).

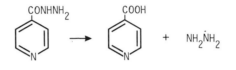

Isoniazid   Isonicotinic Acid   Hydrazine

Figure 4.40. Hydrolysis of isoniazid.

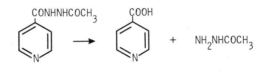

Acetylisoniazid   Isonicotinic Acid   Acetylhydrazine

Figure 4.41. Hydrolysis of acetylisoniazid.

Hydrolysis of carbamates

The insecticide carbaryl is hydrolysed by liver enzymes to 1-naphthol (figure 4.42). This compound also undergoes extensive metabolism by other routes.

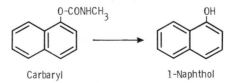

Carbaryl   1-Naphthol

Figure 4.42. Hydrolysis of carbaryl.

Hydration of epoxides

Epoxides, three-membered rings containing an oxygen atom, may be metabolized by the enzyme epoxide hydratase. This enzyme adds water to the epoxide to yield a trans-dihydrodiol (figure 4.43). Epoxides are often intermediates produced by the oxidation of unsaturated double bonds, aromatic, aliphatic or heterocyclic, as for example takes place during the hydroxylation of bromobenzene, the hepatotoxic solvent (figure 7.9).

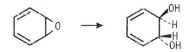

Benzene-1,2-oxide   Benzene trans 1,2-dihydrodiol

Figure 4.43. Hydration of benzene-1,2-oxide by epoxide hydratase.

The enzyme is found in the microsomal fraction of the cell in close proximity to the cytochrome P-450 group of mono-oxygenases. Epoxide hydratase is therefore well placed to carry out its important role in detoxifying the chemically unstable and often toxic epoxide intermediates produced by cytochrome P-450 mediated hydroxylation.

The epoxide of bromobenzene is one such toxic intermediate and this example is discussed in more detail in Chapter 7. In the case of some carcinogenic polycyclic hydrocarbons, however, it seems that the dihydrodiol products are in turn further metabolized to epoxide-diols, the ultimate carcinogens (see page 181).

Phase 2 reactions

Conjugation

Conjugation reactions involve the addition to foreign compounds of endogenous groups which are generally polar and readily available *in vivo*. These groups are added to a suitable functional group present on the foreign molecule or introduced by Phase 1 metabolism. This renders the whole molecule more polar and less lipid-soluble, thus facilitating excretion. The groups donated in conjugation reactions are often involved in intermediary metabolism.

Glucuronide formation

This is a major conjugation reaction occurring in most species and it involves the transfer of glucuronic acid from uridine diphosphate glucuronic acid (UDPGA). The atoms to which glucuronic acid may be attached are oxygen in hydroxyl and carboxyl groups, and in some cases sulphur and nitrogen atoms. The enzymes catalysing the conjugation reactions, the glucuronyl transferases, are found in the microsomal fraction. The donor, UDP-glucuronic acid, is formed in the soluble fraction of hepatic cells from glucose-1-phosphate, as indicated in figure 4.44. UDP-glucuronic acid is able

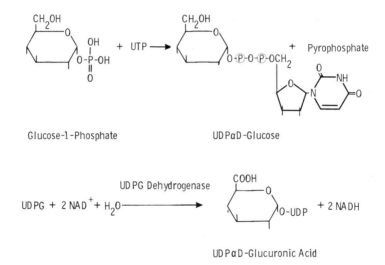

Figure 4.44. Formation of uridine diphosphate glucuronic acid (UDPGA).

to donate glucuronic acid to a wide variety of substrates, including endogenous substances. Conjugation with glucuronic acid involves nucleophilic attack by the oxygen, sulphur or nitrogen atom at the C-1 carbon atom of the glucuronic acid moiety. Glucuronides are therefore generally β in configuration. Conjugation with hydroxyl groups gives ether glucuronides and with carboxylic acids, ester glucuronides (figure 4.45). Amino groups may be conjugated directly, as in the case of aniline (figure 4.46) or through an oxygen atom as in the case of *N*-hydroxy compounds, such as the carcinogen *N*-hydroxyacetylaminofluorene (figure 4.47).

Certain thiols may be conjugated directly through the sulphur atom (figure 4.48).

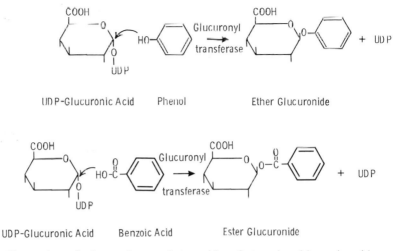

UDP-Glucuronic Acid   Phenol   Ether Glucuronide

UDP-Glucuronic Acid   Benzoic Acid   Ester Glucuronide

Figure 4.45. Formation of ether and ester glucuronides of phenol and benzoic acid respectively.

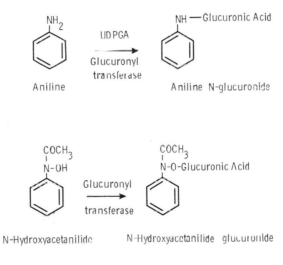

Aniline   Aniline N-glucuronide

N-Hydroxyacetanilide   N-Hydroxyacetanilide glucuronide

Figure 4.46. Glucuronidation of aniline and *N*-hydroxyacetanilide.

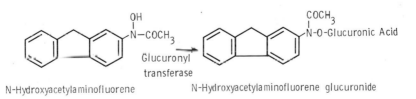

N-Hydroxyacetylaminofluorene   N-Hydroxyacetylaminofluorene glucuronide

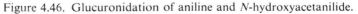

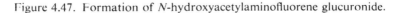

Figure 4.47. Formation of *N*-hydroxyacetylaminofluorene glucuronide.

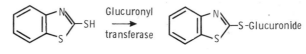

2-Mercaptobenzothiazole   2-Mercaptobenzothiazole-S-glucuronide

Figure 4.48. Formation of 2-mercaptobenzothiazole-S-glucuronide.

Although conjugation generally decreases biological activity, including toxicity, occasionally the latter is increased, as in the case of acetylaminofluorene. The *N*-hydroxyglucuronide is a more potent carcinogen (figure 4.47).

Analogues of purines and pyrimidines may be conjugated with ribose or ribose phosphates to give ribonucleotides and ribonucleosides.

Sulphate conjugation

The formation of sulphate esters is a major route of conjugation for various types of hydroxyl group, and may also occur with amino groups. Thus, substrates include aliphatic alcohols, phenols, aromatic amines and also endogenous compounds such as steroids and carbohydrates (figures 4.49 and 4.50).

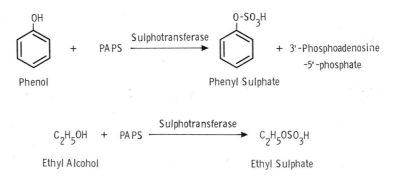

Figure 4.49. Formation of ethereal sulphates of phenol and ethyl alcohol.

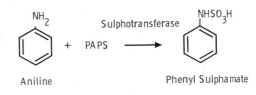

Figure 4.50. Sulphate conjugation of aniline.

The sulphate donor is 3'-phosphoadenosine-5'-phosphosulphate (PAPS), and the conjugation is catalysed by a sulphotransferase (figure 4.51). There are a variety of sulphotransferase enzymes found in the soluble fraction of cells from various tissues, particularly the liver, intestinal mucosa and kidney.

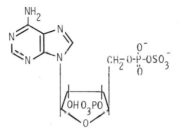

Phosphoadenosinephosphosulphate   PAPS

Figure 4.51. Structure of 3-phosphoadenosine-5'-phosphosulphate (PAPS).

PAPS is formed from inorganic sulphate and ATP. This inorganic sulphate precursor of PAPS may become depleted when large amounts of a foreign compound conjugated with sulphate, such as paracetamol, are administered. Sulphate conjugation may increase toxicity in certain rare cases as with the conjugation of *N*-hydroxyacetylaminofluorene, the carcinogen (see Chapter 7, figure 7.1).

Glutathione conjugation

Certain types of foreign compound are excreted as conjugates with *N*-acetylcysteine (mercapturic acid conjugates). These conjugates generally result from an initial conjugation with glutathione followed by metabolic cleavage of the glutamyl and glycinyl residues and then acetylation of the cysteine moiety. The initial conjugation reactions are catalysed by gluta-thione-*S*-transferases, and there are a variety of these enzymes, each catalysing conjugations with different substrates, both aromatic and aliphatic. The glutathione transferases are primarily found in the soluble fraction of the cell, but are also present in the microsomes.

In many cases the sulphydryl group of glutathione acts as a nucleophile, attacking the reactive electrophilic centre in the foreign molecule. Consequently, conjugation with glutathione is often important toxicologically. There are a variety of substrates for this reaction, the mechanism of which may vary. Thus, aromatic hydrocarbons, alkyl halides, aryl halides, aryl epoxides, alkyl epoxides, aromatic nitro compounds and alkenes may all be conjugated with glutathione and excreted as mercapturic acids. In some cases, enzymic catalysis may not be necessary, a chemical reaction between the activated substrate and glutathione being sufficient.

The conjugation of the aromatic hydrocarbon naphthalene with glutathione has been well characterized and is shown in figure 4.52.

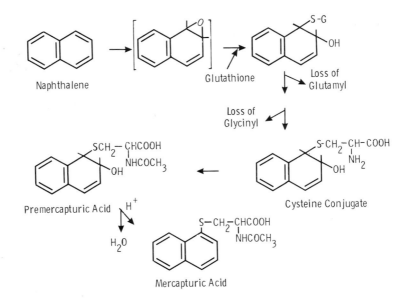

Figure 4.52. Conjugation of naphthalene-1,2-oxide with glutathione and formation of naphthalene mercapturic acid.

Glutathione conjugates may be excreted in the bile unchanged, that is, before further metabolism to mercapturic acids. Intermediates in the degradation of glutathione conjugates such as cysteinyl–glycine conjugates may also be excreted in the bile.

Metabolic activation of aromatic and aliphatic compounds to chemically reactive intermediates may often be followed by glutathione conjugation, effectively a detoxication and removal of a reactive electrophile. This may be one of the numerous functions of glutathione in the cell. In the case of naphthalene metabolism, the activation produces an epoxide (figure 4.52), as is the case with a number of aromatic hydrocarbons, from the simple benzene to the polycyclic benzo[*a*]pyrene, which are excreted as mercapturic acids. Saturated and unsaturated aliphatic compounds may also be metabolized to epoxides and excreted as mercapturic acids as illustrated in figure 4.53.

Alternatively, some halogenated aliphatic compounds may be conjugated with glutathione, leading to a displacement of the halogen (figure 4.54). This reaction may occur by a glutathione transferase-catalysed nucleophilic

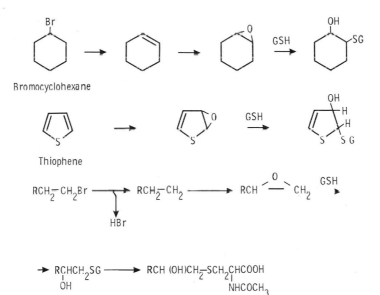

Figure 4.53. Conjugation of various epoxides with glutathione.

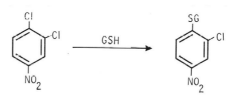

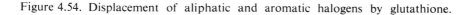

3, 4-Dichloronitrobenzene

Figure 4.54. Displacement of aliphatic and aromatic halogens by glutathione.

substitution. Similarly, halogenated aromatic and nitro compounds are conjugated with glutathione with loss of the halogen or nitro group, as shown in figure 4.54. Some halogenated aromatic compounds may be activated via an epoxide and then conjugated with glutathione, however, such as bromobenzene (see page 194).

Unsaturated aliphatic compounds with suitable electron-withdrawing groups may react directly with glutathione without undergoing metabolic activation. For example, diethyl maleate reacts readily with glutathione *in vivo* (figure 4.55). Diethyl maleate may be used to deplete hepatic glutathione *in vivo* experimentally, as can a number of compounds which are conjugated with the tripeptide, if given in sufficiently large doses.

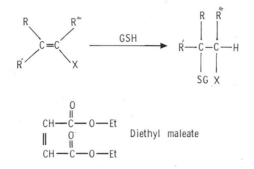

Figure 4.55. Conjugation of an unsaturated aliphatic compound with glutathione and structure of diethyl maleate, a typical example.

Acetylation

Acetylation is an important route of metabolism for aromatic amines, sulphonamides and hydrazines, and there is a wide variety of substrates. The enzyme which catalyses this reaction is an acetyltransferase and it is found in the cytosol of hepatic reticulo-endothelial cells, in the gastrointestinal mucosal cells and also in white blood cells. The enzyme has been purified, its mechanism of action extensively studied and it is now well understood.

The coenzyme utilized in the acetyltransferase-catalysed reactions is acetyl CoA, which transfers the acetyl group to the enzyme which in turn acetylates the substrate, as shown below in figure 4.56.

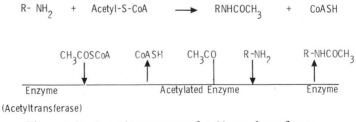

Figure 4.56. Reaction sequence for *N*-acetyltransferase.

A typical substrate is sulphanilamide, which may be acetylated on either the N^4, amino nitrogen or the N^1, sulphonamido nitrogen (figure 4.57).

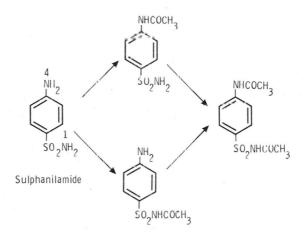

Figure 4.57. Acetylation of sulphanilamide on the N^1-sulphonamido or N^4-amino nitrogen to give the N^1 and N^4-acetyl and N^1,N^4-diacetyl derivatives.

It has been found, however, that the acetylation of certain compounds in man and in the rabbit shows wide interindividual variation. This variation in acetylation has a genetic basis and shows a bimodal distribution, the two phenotypes being termed rapid and slow acetylators. It is probable that in man this polymorphism reflects different forms of the acetyltransferase, as has been shown to be the case in the rabbit.

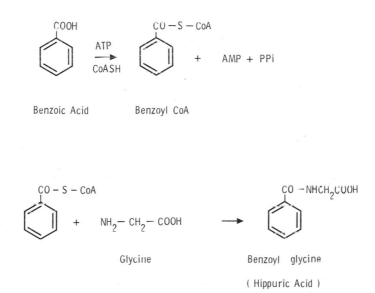

Figure 4.58. Conjugation of benzoic acid with glycine.

The acetylation polymorphism has a number of toxicological consequences which will be discussed more fully in Chapters 5 and 7. Only certain substrates are polymorphically acetylated. Some compounds, notably sulphanilamide, *p*-aminosalicylic acid and *p*-aminobenzoic acid, are monomorphically acetylated (figures 4.57 and 5.11).

Conjugation with amino acids

Foreign compounds containing a carboxylic acid group may be excreted as peptide conjugates. The amino acid most commonly utilized is glycine, but conjugates with ornithine, taurine and glutamine are also known. The reaction involves acylation of the amino group of the amino acid by the foreign carboxylic acid group. The reaction is therefore the converse of acetylation as described above.

The carboxylic acid group is first converted into a CoA derivative which then acylates the amino group as illustrated with benzoic acid (figure 4.58). The acylase enzyme catalysing this reaction is found in liver mitochondria.

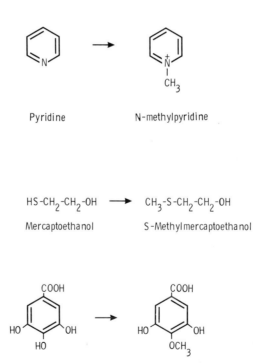

Pyridine   N-methylpyridine

$HS-CH_2-CH_2-OH \longrightarrow CH_3-S-CH_2-CH_2-OH$

Mercaptoethanol   S-Methylmercaptoethanol

3,4,5-Trihydroxybenzoic Acid   3,5-Dihydroxy-4-methoxybenzoic Acid

Figure 4.59. *N, O* and *S* methylation.

Methylation

Amino, hydroxyl and thiol groups in foreign compounds (figure 4.59) may undergo methylation *in vivo*, as do certain endogenous compounds such as catecholamines. The reactions are catalysed by various methyl transferase enzymes. The methyl donor is *S*-adenosyl methionine, which is formed by the reaction of methionine with ATP (see Chapter 7, figure 7.7). The methyl transferases may be found in the soluble fraction of cells from different and in some cases very specific tissues. Certain of these enzymes may also be found in the microsomal fraction.

Catechol and trihydric phenol derivatives may be methylated *in vivo* by transferases found in both soluble and microsomal fractions (figure 4.59). The methyl transferase which catalyses the methylation of thiol groups (figure 4.59) is a microsomal enzyme which is found in a number of tissues.

Bibliography

BRODIE, B. B., GILLETTE, J. R. & ACKERMAN, H. S. (editors) (1971) *Handbook of Experimental Pharmacology*, Vol. 28, Part 2, *Concepts in Biochemical Pharmacology* (Berlin: Springer Verlag). (This volume contains chapters on the major types of metabolic reaction, both phase 1 and phase 2).

CHASSEAUD, L. F. (1976) Conjugation with glutathione and mercapturic acid excretion. In *Glutathione. Metabolism and Function*, edited by I. M. Arias and W. B. Jakoby (New York: Raven Press).

GOLDSTEIN, A., ARONOW, L. & KALMAN, S. M. (1974) Drug metabolism. Chapter 3 of *Principles of Drug Action: The Basis of Pharmacology* (New York: John Wiley).

GRAM, T. E. (editor) (1980) *Extrahepatic Metabolism of Drugs and Other Foreign Compounds* (Jamaica, New York: Spectrum Publications). (This text contains chapters on various aspects of drug metabolism, both phase 1 and phase 2.)

HATHWAY, D. E., BROWN, S. S., CHASSEAUD, L. F. & HUTSON, D. H. (reporters) (1970–1981) *Foreign Compound Metabolism in Mammals*, Vols. 1–6 (London: The Chemical Society).

HODGSON, E. & GUTHRIE, F. E. (editors) (1980) *Introduction to Biochemical Toxicology*, Chapters 5 and 6 (New York: Elsevier-North Holland).

HUCKER, H. B. (1973) Intermediates in drug metabolism reactions. *Drug Metab. Rev.*, **2**, 33.

JENNER, P. & TESTA, B. (1978) Novel pathways in drug metabolism. *Xenobiotica*, **8**, 1.

JERINA, D. M. & DALY, J. W. (1974) Arene oxides: A new aspect of drug metabolism. *Science*, **185**, 573.

JERINA, D. M., DALY, J. W. & WITKOP, B. (1971) The "NIH Shift" and a mechanism of enzymatic oxygenation. In *Biogenic Amines and Physiological Membranes in Drug Therapy*, edited by I. H. Biel and L. G. Abood (New York: Marcel Dekker).

MURPHY, S. D. (1980) Pesticides. In *Cassaret and Doull's Toxicology, The Basic Science of Poisons*, edited by J. Doull, C. D. Klaassen and M. O. Amdur (New York: Macmillan).

OESCH, F. (1972) Mammalian epoxide hydrases: Inducible enzymes catalysing the inactivation of carcinogenic and cytotoxic metabolites derived from aromatic and olefinic compounds. *Xenobiotica*, **3**, 305.

PARKE, D. V. (1968) *The Biochemistry of Foreign Compounds* (Oxford: Pergamon).

WILLIAMS, R. T. (1959) *Detoxication Mechanisms* (London: Chapman & Hall).

Chapter 5

Factors affecting metabolism and disposition

Introduction

In the preceding two chapters, the disposition and metabolism of foreign compounds, as determinants of their toxic responses, were discussed. In this chapter, the influence of various factors on these determinants and therefore on their ultimate toxicity will be dealt with.

It is becoming increasingly apparent that the toxicity of a foreign compound and its mode of expression are dependent on many variables. Apart from large variations in susceptibility between species, within the same species many factors may be involved. The genetic constitution of a particular organism is known to be a major factor in conferring susceptibility to toxicity in some cases. The age of the animal and certain characteristics of its organ systems may also be important internal factors.

External factors such as the dose of the compound or the manner in which it is given, the diet of the animal and other foreign compounds to which it is exposed, are also important for the eventual toxic response. Although some of these factors may be controlled in experimental animals, in the human population they remain and may be extremely important.

For a logical use of experimental animals as models for man in toxicity testing, therefore, these factors must be appreciated and utilized for the fullest possible exploration of potential toxicity.

Species

There are many different examples of species differences in the toxicity of foreign compounds, some of which are commercially useful to man, as in the case of pesticides and antibiotic drugs. These differences may be related to differences in the metabolism and disposition of such compounds, and may be extremely important in toxicity testing and in the useful exploitation of selective toxicity.

Species differences in disposition

Absorption

Absorption of foreign compounds from various sites is dependent on the physiological and physical conditions at these sites. These, of course, may be subject to species variations. Absorption of compounds through the skin shows considerable species variation. Table 5.1 gives an example of this and shows the species differences in toxicity of an organophosphorus compound absorbed percutaneously.

Table 5.1. Species differences in the relative percutaneous toxicity and skin penetration of organophosphorus compounds.

Species	Rate ($\mu g/cm^2$)/min	Compound 1†	Compound 2†	2/1
Pig	0·3	10·0	80·0	8·0
Dog	2·7	1·9	10·8	5·7
Monkey	4·2	4·4	13·0	3·0
Goat	4·4	3·0	4·0	1·3
Cat	4·4	0·9	2·4	2·7
Rabbit	9·3	1·0	5·0	5·0
Rat	9·3	17·0	20·0	1·2
Mouse	—	6·0	9·2	1·5
Guinea-pig	6·0	—	—	—

† Values are expressed as the ratio of the LD_{50} of that compound to the rabbit LD_{50} of compound 1.
Data from McCreesh (1965) *Toxic. appl. Pharmac.*, Suppl. 2, **7**, 20, and Adamson & Davies (1973). In *International Encyclopaedia of Pharmacology and Therapeutics*, Section 85, Chapter 9 (Oxford: Pergamon).

Oral absorption depends partially on the pH of the gastrointestinal tract. It is known that the environment of the gastrointestinal tract varies with species, as shown in table 5.2. Obviously, considerable differences in the absorption of weak acids from the stomach may occur between species. Similarly, differences might be seen in compounds which are susceptible to

Table 5.2. Species differences in pH of saliva and gastric juices.

Species	pH (Saliva)	pH (Gastric juice)
Man	6·75	1·5–2·5
Dog	7·5	1·5–2·0[1]
		4·5[2]
Cat	7·5	
Rat	8·2–8·9	2·0–4·0
Horse	7·3–8·6	4·46
Cattle	8·1–8·8	5·5–6·5
Sheep	8·4–8·7	7·6–8·?
Chicken		4·2
Frog		2·2–3·7

[1] Fasting; [2] Fed.

Data from Altman & Dittmer (1961) *Blood and Other Body Fluids* (Washington D.C.: Federation of American Societies for Experimental Biology); Dobson (1967) *Fed. Proc.*, **26**, 994; Levine (1965) *Life Sci.*, **4**, 959; Prosser & Brown (1961) *Comparative Animal Physiology* (Philadelphia: W. B. Saunders); Bishop *et al.* (1950) *Comparative Animal Physiology* (Philadelphia: W. B. Saunders).

the acidic conditions of the stomach, such that a foreign compound would be more stable in the gastric juice of a sheep than that of a rat. For instance, the difference in acute toxicity of pyrvinium chloride after oral but not intraperitoneal administration between rats and mice is apparently due to the difference in absorption from the gastrointestinal tract.

Distribution

The distribution of foreign compounds may vary between species because of differences in a number of factors. For instance, differences in localization of methylglyoxal-bis-guanyl hydrazone (figure 5.1) in the liver accounts for its

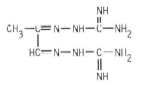

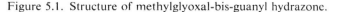

Figure 5.1. Structure of methylglyoxal-bis-guanyl hydrazone.

Table 5.3. Binding of various sulphonamides to plasma of various species.

Sulphonamide	Percent bound at concentration of 100 µg/ml							
	Human	Monkey	Dog	Cat	Mouse	Chicken	Bovine plasma	Bovine albumin
Sulphadiazine	33	35	17	13	7	16	24	24
Sulphamethoxypyridazine	83	81	60	49	28	14	66	60
Sulphisoxazole	84	86	68	43	31	5	76	76
Sulphaethylthiadiazole	95	90	86	76	38	48	87	87

Data from Adamson & Davies (1973). In *International Encyclopaedia of Pharmacology and Therapeutics*, Section 85, Chapter 9 (Oxford: Pergamon).

greater hepatotoxicity in rats than in mice. The hepatic concentration in mice is only 0·3–0·5 % of the dose after 48 hours, compared with 2–8 % in the rat.

The plasma protein concentration is a species-dependent variable, and the proportions and types of proteins may also vary. The concentration may vary from about 20 g/l in certain fish to 83 g/l in cattle. Thus, foreign compounds may bind to plasma proteins to very different extents in different species (table 5.3). Because the extent of binding may be a very important determinant of the free concentration of a compound in the plasma and the tissues, this species difference may be an important determinant of toxicity. The free form of the compound is the important moiety as far as toxicity is concerned.

The distribution of foreign compounds may also depend on their metabolism, the rate of which may determine the rate of removal from the plasma or the rate of excretion and hence the tissue and plasma concentration. Therefore, species differences in metabolism may also be important factors.

Excretion

Renal excretion. Although most mammals have similar kidneys, there are functional differences between species and urine pH, and volume and rate of production may vary considerably (table 5.4). Thus, the rate of urine production in the rat is an order of magnitude greater than the rate in man. Although

Table 5.4. Variation in urinary volume and pH with species.

Species	Volume (ml/kg)/day	pH
Man	9–29	6·3 (4·8–7·8)
Monkey	70–80	—
Dog	20–100	5·0–7·0
Cat	10–20	5·0–7·0
Rabbit	50–75	—
Rat	150–300	—
Horse	3–18	7–8
Cattle	17–45	7–8
Sheep	10–40	7–8
Swine	5–30	Acid or Alkaline

Data from Altman & Dittmer (1961) *Blood and Other Body Fluids* (Washington D.C.: Federation of American Societies for Experimental Biology); Bloom (1960) *The Urine of the Dog and Cat* (New York: Gamma Publications); Cornelius & Kaneko (1963) *Clinical Biochemistry of Domestic Animals* (New York: Academic Press).

D

the pH ranges for the urine of a number of mammals may overlap (table 5.4), a small change in pH may markedly change the solubility of a foreign compound and therefore its excretion. For instance, some of the sulphona-mides and their acetylated metabolites show marked changes in solubility for a pH change of one unit (table 4.1), and renal toxicity due to crystallization of the drug or its metabolites in the renal tubules has been known to occur when high doses are used. The species differences in renal excretion for an unmetabolized compound, methylglyoxal-bis-guanylhydrazone, are shown in table 5.5, and it can be seen that the rat excretes twice the amount excreted by man in 24 hours.

Table 5.5 Urinary excretion of methylglyoxal-bis-guanylhydra-zone in mammalian species.

Species	Dose (mg/kg)	Percent excreted	Time period for excretion (h)
Mouse	20 (i.v.)	51	24
Rat	20 (i.p.)	65	24
Dog	20 (i.v.)	26	24
		52	48
		66	96
Monkey	25 (i.v.)	47	24
Man	4 (i.v.)	25	24
		42	118
		49	166

Data from Oliverio *et al.* (1963) *J. Pharmac. exp. Ther.*, **141**, 149; Adamson & Davies (1973). In *International Encyclopaedia of Pharmacology and Therapeutics*, Section 85, Chapter 9 (Oxford: Pergamon).

Biliary excretion. The extent of excretion of foreign compounds via the bile is influenced by a number of factors, the molecular weight of the compound being the major one. However, the molecular weight threshold for biliary excretion may show considerable species differences. Little biliary excretion (5–10% of the dose) occurs for compounds of molecular weight of less than 300. Above this value, however, the bile may become a major route of elimination, and it is probably around this value that species variations are most noticeable. Thus, for methylene di-salicylic acid (mol. wt. 288), the dog excretes 65% in the bile, whereas the guinea-pig excretes only 4% (table 5.6). Similarly, the biliary excretion of succinyl sulphathiazole (mol. wt. 355) shows more than a tenfold variation between the rhesus monkey and the rat (table 5.6).

Table 5.6. Biliary excretion of compounds of molecular size 300–500 in various species.

	Percent dose excreted in bile				
	Methylenedisalicylic acid (mol. wt. 288, 20 mg/kg, i.v., 6 h)	Succinylsulpha-thiazole (mol. wt. 355, 20 mg/kg, i.v., 6 h)	Stilboestrol glucuronide (mol. wt. 445, 10 mg/kg, i.v., 3 h)	Sulphadimethoxine-N^1-glucuronide (mol. wt. 487, 15 mg/kg, i.v., 3 h)	Phenolphthalein glucuronide (mol. wt. 495, 10 mg/kg, i.v., 3 h)
Rhesus monkey	—	0·2	—	—	9
Rat	54	29	95	43	54
Hen	—	25	—	—	—
Dog	65	20	65	43	81
Cat	—	7	77	—	34
Sheep	—	7	—	—	38
Rabbit	5	1	32	10	13
Guinea-pig	4	1	20	12	6
Pig	—	0·2	—	—	—

Data from Abou-El-Makarem *et al.* (1967) *Biochem. J.*, **105**, 1289, and Davison & Williams (1968) *J. Pharm. Pharmac.*, **20**, 12.

The species pattern of the rabbit and the guinea-pig being poor biliary excretors and the rat being an extensive biliary excretor is maintained with many other compounds. With compounds of higher molecular weight, however, species differences are less, as illustrated by the compound indocyanine green (table 5.7). The metabolism of a compound obviously influences the extent of biliary excretion, and therefore species differences in metabolism may also be a factor.

Table 5.7. Biliary excretion of indocyanine green in various species.

Species	Dose (mg/kg, i.v.)	% Dose in bile†
Rat	0·5	60
Rat	2·5	82
Dog	1–7	97
Rabbit	2·5	94
Man	0·5	High
Man	2·0	High

† Excreted unchanged.
Data from Caesar *et al.* (1961) *Clin. Sci.*, **21**, 43; Cherrick *et al.* (1960) *J. clin Invest.*, **39**, 592; Delaney *et al.* (1969) unpublished data; Levine *et al.* (1970) *Biochem. Pharmac.*, **19**, 235; Wheeler *et al.* (1958) *Proc. Soc. exp. Biol. Med. N.Y.*, **99**, 11.

The rate of bile secretion and the pH of the bile may also be determinants of the extent of biliary excretion of a foreign compound, and these also show species variations. The fate of compounds excreted in the bile may also depend on the species, as differences in intestinal pH and flora occur. A particularly important consequence of biliary excretion is metabolism by the gut flora and reabsorption. This enterohepatic circulation prolongs the length of time the animal is exposed to the foreign compound, and may introduce novel toxic metabolites. This could therefore result in marked species differences in toxicity.

Species differences in metabolism

Although certain types of metabolic reaction are known to be absent from particular species, in general there is no apparent pattern in evolutionary development. Thus, bacteria are capable of carrying out many different types of biotransformation.

Examples of toxicologically important species differences in metabolism will therefore be dealt with by considering the different types of metabolic reactions.

Phase I reactions

Oxidation. Although most of the common mammals used as experimental animals carry out oxidation reactions, there may be large variations in the extent to which some of these are carried out. The most common species differences are in the rate at which a particular compound is oxidized rather than the particular pathway through which it is metabolized. Most species are able to hydroxylate aromatic compounds, but there is no apparent species pattern in the ability to carry out this metabolic transformation.

Fish have a relatively poor ability for oxidative metabolism compared with the commonly used laboratory animals such as rats and mice. Insects such as flies have microsomal enzymes, and these are involved in the metabolism of the insecticide parathion to the more toxic paraoxon as discussed in the previous chapter (figure 4.23).

However, there are known instances of differences in the preferred route of metabolism which are important in toxicity, as well as simple differences in the route of a particular oxidation. For example, the oxidative metabolism of ethylene glycol gives rise to either carbon dioxide or oxalic acid (figure 5.2). The relative importance of these two pathways is reflected in the toxicity. Thus, the production of oxalic acid is in the order: cat > rat > rabbit, and this is also the order of increasing toxicity (figure 5.3). The aromatic hydroxylation of aniline (figure 5.4) shows marked species differences in the position of substitution, as shown in table 5.8. The preferred route of hydroxylation also correlates with the toxicity, such that those species to which aniline is particularly toxic, such as the cat and dog, produce mainly *o*-aminophenol, whereas those producing *p*-aminophenol, such as the rat and hamster, seem less susceptible. Conversely, the hydroxylation of coumarin at the seven position (figure 4.14) is an important pathway in the rabbit and also the

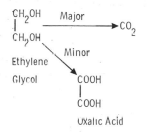

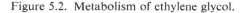

Figure 5.2. Metabolism of ethylene glycol.

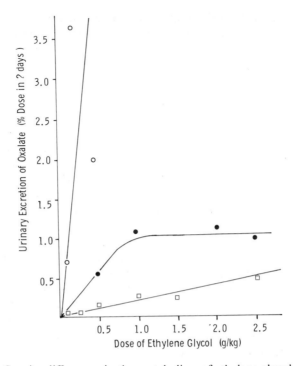

Figure 5.3. Species differences in the metabolism of ethylene glycol to oxalate after increasing doses. Species used were cats (○), rats (●) and rabbits (□). Data from Gessner *et al.* (1961) *Biochem. J.*, **79**, 482. Adapted from Parke, D. V. (1968) *The Biochemistry of Foreign Compounds* (Oxford: Pergamon).

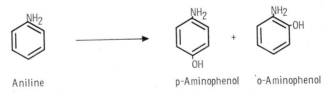

Figure 5.4. Aromatic hydroxylation of aniline.

hamster and cat, but not in the rat or mouse. It is clear that, even with aromatic hydroxylation, species cannot be readily grouped.

The *N*-hydroxylation of acetylaminofluorene and paracetamol are two toxicologically important examples illustrating species differences (see Chapter 7). Another example is the metabolism of amphetamine, which reveals marked species differences in the preferred route, as shown in figure 5.5.

Species differences in the rate of metabolism of hexobarbital *in vitro* correlate with the plasma half-life and duration of action *in vivo* as shown in table 5.9. This data shows that the marked differences in enzyme activity

Table 5.8. Species differences in the hydroxylation of aniline.

Species	% Dose excreted	
	o-Aminophenol	*p*-Aminophenol
Gerbil	3	48
Guinea-pig	4	46
Golden hamster	6	53
Chicken	11	44
Rat	19	48
Ferret	26	28
Dog	18	9
Cat	32	14

Data from Parke, D. V. (1968) *The Biochemistry of Foreign Compounds* (Oxford: Pergamon).

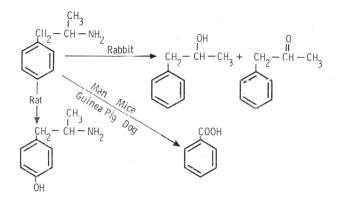

Figure 5.5. Species differences in the metabolism of amphetamine.

between species is the major determinant of the biological activity in this case.

A recent example of a species difference in metabolism causing a difference in toxicity is afforded by the alicyclic hydroxylation of an oral anti-allergy drug (FPL57787; figure 5.6). After chronic administration this compound was found to be hepatotoxic in dogs but not in rats. It was found that dogs did not significantly metabolize the compound by alicyclic oxidation, whereas rats, hamsters, rabbits and man excreted substantial proportions of metabolites in the urine. In the dog, biliary excretion was the route of elimination of the unchanged compound, and after toxic doses were administered, this route was saturated. Hence, the toxicity was probably due to the accumulation of high levels of the unchanged compound.

Table 5.9. Species differences in the duration of action and metabolism of hexobarbital (dose of barbiturate 100 mg/kg (50 mg/kg in dogs)).

Species	Duration of action (min)	Plasma half-life (min)	Relative enzyme activity ($(\mu g/g)/h$)	Plasma level on awakening ($\mu g/ml$)
Mouse	12	19	598	89
Rabbit	49	60	196	57
Rat	90	140	135	64
Dog	315	260	36	19

Data from Quinn *et al.* (1958) *Biochem. Pharmac.*, **1**, 152.

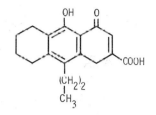

Figure 5.6. Structure of FPL 57787.

Hydrolytic reactions. There are numerous different esterases responsible for the hydrolysis of esters and amides, and they occur in most species. However, the activity may vary considerably between species. For example, the insecticide malathion owes its selective toxicity to this difference. In mammals, the major route of metabolism is hydrolysis to the dicarboxylic acid, whereas in insects it is oxidation to malaoxon (figure 5.7). Malaoxon is a very potent cholinesterase inhibitor, and its insecticidal action is probably due to this property. The hydrolysis product has a low mammalian toxicity (see Chapter 7).

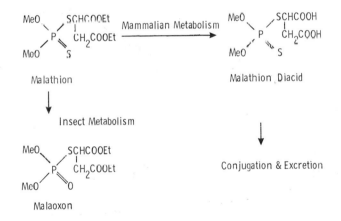

Figure 5.7. Metabolism of malathion.

Another example is dimethoate, the toxicity of which is related to its rate of hydrolysis. Those species which are capable of metabolizing the insecticide are less susceptible than those species which are poor metabolizers. The metabolism of dimethoate is shown in figure 5.8. Studies on the metabolism *in vitro* of dimethoate have shown that sheep liver produces only the first metabolite, whereas guinea-pigs produce only the final product (figure 5.8). Rats and mice metabolize dimethoate to both products. The toxicity is in the descending order—sheep > dog > rat > cattle > guinea-pig > mouse.

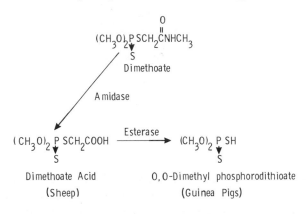

Figure 5.8. Metabolism of dimethoate.

Reduction. The activity of azo and nitroreductase varies between different species, as shown by the *in vitro* data in table 5.10. Thus, azoreductase activity is particularly high in the guinea-pig, relative to the other species studied, whereas nitroreductase activity is greatest in the mouse liver.

Phase II reactions

Species vary considerably in the extent to which they conjugate foreign compounds, but this is generally a quantitative rather than a qualitative difference. Thus, most species have a preferred route of conjugation but other routes are still available and utilized.

Table 5.10. Hepatic azoreductase and nitroreductase activities of various species.

Species (male)	Azoreductase (μmol sulphanilamide formed per g liver per h)	Nitroreductase (μmol *p*-aminobenzoic acid formed per g liver per h)
Mouse	6·7–9·6[1]	2·1–3·2[1]
Rat	5·9	2·1
Guinea-pig	9·0	2·0
Pigeon	7·1	1·1
Turtle	1·4 (0·5)[2]	0·15 (2·5)[2]
Frog	1·2 (0·6)[2]	0 (0)[2]

[1] According to strain.

[2] Temperature of incubation 21 °C (temperature elsewhere 37 °C).

Substrates used were neoprontosil for the azoreductase and *p*-nitrobenzoic acid for the nitroreductase.

Data from Adamson *et al*. (1965) *Proc. natn. Acad. Sci.*, **54**, 1386.

Glucuronide conjugation. Conjugation of foreign compounds with glucuronic acid is an important route of metabolism in most animals, namely mammals, birds, amphibians and reptiles, but not fish. In insects, glucoside conjugates utilizing glucose rather than glucuronic acid are formed. The major exception with regard to glycoside conjugation is the cat, which is virtually unable to form glucuronides of certain foreign compounds. This is due to a deficiency in the enzyme glucuronyl transferase. However, bilirubin glucuronide is formed in the cat, suggesting that this requires a different enzyme. The cat is therefore more susceptible to the toxic effects of phenols than species able to detoxify them by glucuronide conjugation.

Sulphate conjugation. Conjugation of foreign compounds with sulphate occurs in most mammals, amphibians, birds, reptiles and insects, but, as with glucuronidation, not in fish. The pig, however, has a reduced ability to form certain ethereal sulphate conjugates, such as with phenol, whereas 1-naphthol is excreted as a sulphate conjugate.

Conjugation with amino acids. Considerable species differences exist in the conjugation of aromatic carboxylic acids with amino acids. A number of amino acids may be utilized, although conjugation with glycine is the most common route (figure 4.58) and occurs in most species except some birds, where ornithine is the preferred amino acid. Certain species also employ glutamine and taurine for conjugation, reptiles may excrete ornithine conjugates as well as glycine conjugates, and some insects utilize mainly arginine.

Aromatic acids may also be excreted as glucuronic acid conjugates, and the relative importance of glucuronic acid conjugation versus amino acid conjugation depends on the particular species and the structure of the compound. Herbivores generally favour amino acid conjugation, carnivores favour glucuronide formation, and omnivores, such as man, utilize both routes of metabolism.

There are also species differences in the site of conjugation; this usually occurs in both liver and kidney, but dogs and chickens carry out this conjugation only in the kidney.

Glutathione conjugation. Conjugation with glutathione, which results in the urinary excretion of *N*-acetylcysteine or cysteine derivatives (figure 4.52) occurs in man, rats, hamsters, mice, dogs, cats, rabbits and guinea-pigs. Guinea-pigs are unusual, however, in generally not excreting *N*-acetylcysteine conjugates, as the enzyme responsible for the acetylation of cysteine is lacking.

Insects are also capable of forming glutathione conjugates, this being probably involved in the dehydrochlorination of the insecticide DDT, a reaction at least some insects, such as flies, are able to carry out (figure 4.36).

Methylation. Methylation of oxygen, sulphur and nitrogen atoms seems to occur in most species of mammal and in those birds, amphibia and insects which have been studied.

Acetylation. Most mammalian species are able to acetylate aromatic amino compounds, the major exception being the dog. Thus, for a number of amino compounds such as procainamide (figure 4.38), sulphadimethoxine, sulphamethomidine, sulphasomizole and the N^4 amino group of sulphanil-amide (figure 4.57), the dog does not excrete the acetylated product. However, the dog does have a high level of deacetylase in the liver and also seems to have an acetyltransferase inhibitor in the liver and kidney. Consequently, acetylation may not be absent in the dog, but rather the products may be hydrolysed or the reaction effectively inhibited.

The dog does, however, acetylate the N^1, sulphonamido group of sulphanilamide (figure 4.57), and also acetylates aliphatic amino groups. The guinea-pig is unable to acetylate aliphatic amino groups such as that in cysteine. Consequently, it excretes cysteine rather than N-acetylcysteine conjugates or mercapturic acids. Birds, some amphibia and insects are able to acetylate aromatic amines, but reptiles do not utilize this reaction.

Concluding remarks

Most species differences in metabolism are quantitative rather than quali-tative; only occasionally does a particular single species show an inability to carry out a particular reaction, or to be its sole exponent. The more common quantitative differences depend on species differences in the enzyme concen-tration or its kinetic parameters, the availability of cofactors and the concentration of substrate in the tissue.

These quantitative differences may often mean, however, that different metabolic routes are favoured in different species, with a consequent differ-ence in pharmacological or toxicological activity.

In general, man is able to carry out all the metabolic transformations found in other mammals and does not show any particular differences in the pres-ence or absence of an enzymatic pathway.

Strain

Differences in the disposition of foreign compounds between different strains of the same species have been documented. For example, mice of various strains show marked differences in the duration of action of hexo-barbital, whereas within any one strain the response is uniform (table 5.11).

Table 5.11 Strain differences in the duration of action of hexobarbital in mice (dose of barbiturate 125 mg/kg body weight).

Strain	Numbers of animals	Mean sleeping time (min) $\pm$ S.D.
A/NL	25	48 ± 4
BALB/cAnN	63	41 ± 2
C57L/HeN	29	33 ± 3
C3HfB/HeN	30	22 ± 3
SWR/HeN	38	18 ± 4
Swiss (non-inbred)	47	43 ± 15

Data from *Jay* (1955) *Proc. Soc. exp. Biol. Med.*, **90**, 378.

The metabolism of antipyrine in rats varies widely between different strains. A well known example of a strain difference is that of the Gunn rat, which is unable to form *o*-glucuronides of bilirubin and most other foreign compounds. This defect is due to a deficiency in glucuronyl transferase. *N*-acetyltransferase activity has been found to vary with the strain of rats and mice. The hydrolysis of acetylisoniazid to acetylhydrazine (figure 4.41) was found to be significantly different between two strains of rats, as was the hepatotoxicity of the acetylisoniazid, being greater in the strain with the greater acylamidase activity.

Sex

There are a number of documented differences in the disposition of foreign compounds which are related to the sex of the animal. For instance, the hexobarbital-induced sleeping time is longer in female than in male rats. This is in accord with the view that, in general, male rats metabolize foreign compounds more rapidly than females. Thus, the biological half-life of hexobarbital is considerably longer in female than in male rats, and *in vitro*, the liver microsomal fraction metabolizes both hexobarbital and aminopyrine more rapidly when derived from male rather than female rats. As well as these reactions catalysed by cytochrome P-450, glucuronic acid conjugation is similarly affected, being greater in male than in female microsomes, and the acetylation of sulphanilamide (figure 4.57) is greater in male rats. Sex differences in metabolism depend on the substrate, however. For example, the hydroxylation of aniline or zoxazolamine shows little difference between the sexes, in contrast to the threefold greater metabolism of hexobarbital or aminopyrine in male compared to female rats.

These sex differences, which are less apparent in other species, are probably mainly due to the influence of sex hormones, as the differences appear at puberty and administration of androgens to female rats abolishes the sex differences in enzyme activity. As already mentioned, the pharmacological activity of certain drugs is lengthened in the female rat, and also the toxicity of certain compounds may be increased. Procaine is hydrolysed more in male rats (figure 4.38), with consequently a lower toxicity in this sex, whereas the insecticides aldrin and heptachlor are metabolized more rapidly to the more toxic epoxides in males and are therefore less toxic to females (figure 5.9).

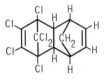

Aldrin

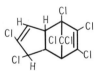

Heptachlor

Figure 5.9. Structures of the insecticides aldrin and heptachlor.

Probably the best example of a sex difference in toxicity is that of the renal toxicity of chloroform in mice. The males are markedly more sensitive than the females, and this difference can be removed by castration of the male animals, and subsequently restored by administration of androgens. Male mice given hexobarbital metabolize it more slowly and the pharmacological effect is more prolonged than in females. The excretion of the food additive butylated hydroxytoluene (figure 5.10) shows an interesting sex difference in rats, being mainly via the urine for males but predominantly via faecal excretion in females, which probably reflects differences in the rates of production of glucuronide and mercapturate conjugates between the sexes.

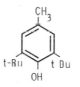

Figure 5.10. Structure of the food additive butylated hydroxytoluene.

Genetic factors

Inherited differences in the metabolism and disposition of foreign compounds which may be seen as strain differences in animals, and as racial and interindividual variability in man, are of great importance in toxicology.

There are many examples of human subjects showing idiosyncratic reactions to the pharmacological or toxicological actions of drugs. In some cases, the genetic basis of such reactions has been established and these cases underline the need for an understanding and appreciation of genetic factors and their role in the causation of toxicity.

It is clear that genetic factors may influence both the response to a toxic compound and the disposition of that compound. For example, in man, deficiency of red cell glucose-6-phosphate dehydrogenase is a genetically determined trait, which is particularly common in certain races. This deficiency results in sensitivity to the acute haemolytic effects of a number of different drugs and compounds, such as primaquine and phenylhydrazine. The red cell is deficient in reduced glutathione and is therefore unable to protect itself from a toxic insult (see page 173). Here, the genetic factor affects the response rather than the disposition.

Genetically determined enzyme deficiencies may of course affect the disposition of the compound rather than the response, and the example of the Gunn rat, which is deficient in glucuronyl transferase, has already been mentioned. Similar defects have been described in man; for example Gilbert's syndrome and the Crigler–Najjar syndrome are both associated with reduced glucuronyl transferase and the consequent reduced ability to conjugate bilirubin. The administration of drugs also conjugated as glucuronides and therefore in competition with the enzyme may lead to blood levels of unconjugated bilirubin sufficient to result in brain damage.

Perhaps one of the best known and fully described genetic factors in drug disposition and metabolism is the acetylator phenotype. It has long been known that some drugs which are acetylated such as isoniazid and procainamide (figures 7.11 and 5.11) show a wide variation in the extent of this acetylation in man and also in the rabbit. This variation shows a bimodal

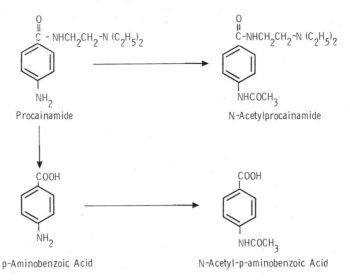

Figure 5.11. Metabolism of procainamide. Procainamide and the hydrolysis product *p*-aminobenzoic acid are both acetylated.

distribution, with subjects falling into slow or rapid acetylator phenotype groups depending on the amount and rate of acetylation (figure 5.12a).

The acetylator phenotype is inherited in the simple Mendelian fashion, being a single gene trait, with two alleles, one for fast acetylation and one for slow acetylation. The allele for slow acetylation is recessive. Therefore, fast acetylators may be homozygous or heterozygous and the slow acetylators only homozygous for the respective alleles.

This genetic trait, which governs the form of *N*-acetyltransferase enzyme present *in vivo*, is found to vary widely in man with the racial origin of the subject. Thus, Egyptians are mainly slow acetylators, whereas Eskimos are almost exclusively rapid acetylators (table 5.12). The acetylation polymorphism is an important genetic factor in a number of toxic reactions (table 5.13). Thus, the slow acetylator phenotype is generally more susceptible than the rapid acetylator, and examples of this are discussed in Chapter 7. However, some foreign compounds are not polymorphically acetylated, for example sulphanilamide, *p*-aminobenzoic acid and *p*-aminosalicyclic acid (figures 4.57 and 5.11), suggesting that other acetyltransferases may be present *in vivo* and involved in the acetylation of these substrates. This is illustrated by the metabolism of procainamide (figure 5.11). The parent compound is polymorphically acetylated (figure 5.12a), whereas the hydrolysis product, *p*-aminobenzoic acid is monomorphically acetylated in the same individuals (figure 5.12b). Although the rabbit is the only other species to show the polymorphism, strain differences in various acetyltransferases have been recently reported in mice and rats.

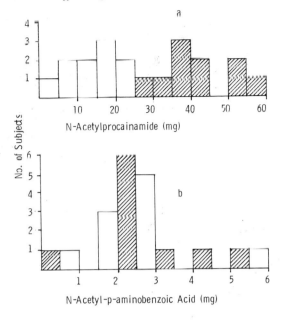

Slow acetylators □   Rapid acetylators ▨

Figure 5.12. Frequency distribution for the acetylation of procainamide (*a*) and *p*-aminobenzoic acid (*b*) in human subjects. Data represents excretion of acetylated product in the urine 6 h after dosing. Data from De Souich & Erill (1976) *Eur. J. clin. Pharm.*, **10**, 283.

Table 5.12. Acetylator phenotype distribution in various ethnic groups (INH, Isoniazid; SMZ, Sulphamethazine).

Ethnic Group	Rapid acetylators (%)	Drug
Eskimos	95–100	INH
Japanese	88	INH
Latin Americans	70	INH
Black Americans	52	INH
White Americans	48	INH
Africans	43	SMZ
South Indians	39	INH
Britons	38	SMZ
Egyptians	18	INH

Data from Lunde *et al.* (1977) *Clin. Pharmacokin.*, **2**, 182.

Table 5.13. Drug toxicities related to the acetylator phenotype.

Drug	Adverse effect	Incidence
Isoniazid	Peripheral neuropathy	Higher in slow acetylators
Isoniazid	Hepatic damage	Higher in rapid acetylators
Procainamide ⎫ Hydralazine ⎭	Lupus erythematosus	Mainly in slow acetylators
Phenelzine	Drowsiness/nausea	More common in slow acetylators

The acetylation polymorphism therefore influences the metabolism of a number of aromatic amines and also their disposition *in vivo*. For example, the plasma half-life of isoniazid is two to three times longer in the slow acetylator than in the rapid acetylator.

Genetic influences are also apparent in oxidation pathways of metabolism, although only recently has this begun to be fully investigated. Early reports of the defective metabolism of diphenylhydantoin in three families and of the defective de-ethylation of phenacetin in certain members of one family indicated a possible genetic component in microsomal enzyme-mediated reactions. Both these cases resulted in enhanced toxicity. Thus, diphenylhydantoin, a commonly used anticonvulsant, normally undergoes aromatic hydroxylation and the corresponding phenolic metabolite is excreted as a glucuronide (figure 7.21). Deficient hydroxylation results in prolonged high blood levels of diphenylhydantoin and the development of toxic effects, such as nystagmus, ataxia and dysarthria. The deficiency in the ability to hydroxylate diphenylhydantoin is inherited with dominant transmission.

The defective de-ethylation of phenacetin was discovered in a patient suffering methaemoglobinaemia after a reasonably small dose of the drug. This toxic effect was observed in a sister of the patient but not in other members of the family. The metabolism of phenacetin in the patient and in the sister was found to involve the production of large amounts of the normally minor metabolites 2-hydroxyphenacetin and 2-hydroxyphenetidine, with a concomitant reduction in the excretion of paracetamol, the major metabolic product of de-ethylation in normal individuals (figure 5.13). It was suggested that autosomal recessive inheritance was involved, with the 2-hydroxylated metabolites probably responsible for the methaemoglobinaemia.

The most recent demonstration of the genetic variability in drug oxidation is provided by the drug debrisoquine (figure 5.14). The alicyclic oxidation of this antihypertensive drug is defective in about 6–8 % of the white Caucasian

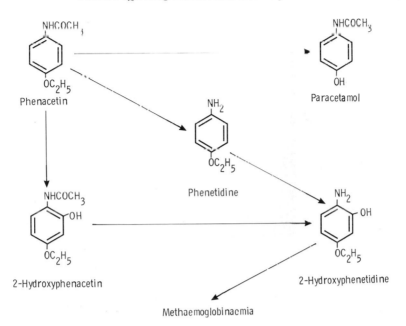

Figure 5.13. Metabolism of phenacetin.

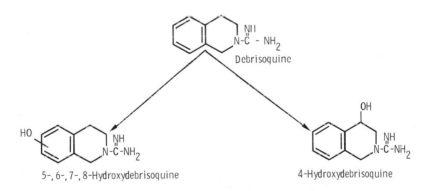

Figure 5.14. Metabolism of debrisoquine in man.

population. This defect is a recessive trait giving rise to a bimodal distribution of oxidative capacity (figure 5.15). The defective hydroxylation is associated with a heightened sensitivity to the hypotensive effect of the drug, and consequently adverse effects follow the normal therapeutic dose in deficient individuals. This deficiency is not restricted to alicyclic oxidation in these individuals, but the aromatic hydroxylation of guanoxon (figure 5.16) and the *o*-de-ethylation of phenacetin are also defective (figure 5.13). The underlying biochemical basis for this polymorphism is not yet clear, but may well

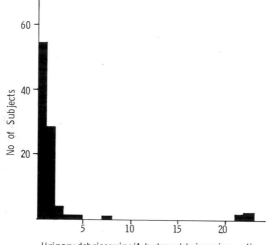

Figure 5.15. Frequency distribution for the ratio urinary debrisoquine : 4-hydroxydebrisoquine in human subjects. Data from Magoub *et al.* (1977) *Lancet*, **2**, 584.

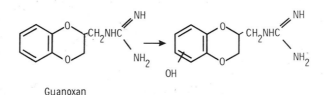

Figure 5.16. Aromatic hydroxylation of guanoxan.

reflect the relative amounts of the various cytochromes P-450 in the liver, in a similar manner to the acetylation polymorphism postulated to involve different acetyltransferase enzymes.

Hydrolysis reactions may also exhibit genetic influences such as the plasma cholinesterase responsible for the metabolism and inactivation of the drug succinylcholine (figure 7.22). Certain individuals may be defective in the ability to hydrolyse and therefore inactivate this drug. Such individuals have a form of the enzyme with a decreased hydrolytic capacity, and they may be affected by the drug for 2–3 hours instead of the more normal two minutes. Apnea may result from the prolonged neuromuscular blockade and muscular relaxation due to the drug. The atypical pseudocholinesterase is inherited as a recessive trait. There are in fact a number of variants of this atypical enzyme which can be differentiated by their sensitivity to certain inhibitors.

Environmental factors

There are many factors in the environment which may influence drug disposition and metabolism and toxicity to a greater or lesser extent. However, as the influence of certain foreign compounds, both drugs and those in the environment, on microsomal enzymes has been well studied, this will constitute a separate section (page 117).

Stress

Adverse environmental conditions or stimuli which create stress in an animal may influence drug metabolism and disposition. Cold stress, for instance, increases aromatic hydroxylation, as does stress due to excessive noise.

Diet

The influence of diet on drug metabolism, disposition and toxicity consists of many constituent factors. Food additives and naturally occurring contaminants in food may influence the activities of various enzymes by induction or inhibition. However, these factors are discussed in a later section (page 117). The factors with which this section will be concerned are the nutritional aspects of diet.

The multitude of factors contained within the environment which may influence drug disposition and metabolism are difficult to separate. The finding that race and diet may affect the clearance of drugs such as antipyrine is such an example. Thus, meat-eating Caucasians have a significantly greater clearance and a shorter plasma half-life for antipyrine than Asian vegetarians. However, the relative importance of race versus diet as contributions to those differences is not clear.

The nutritional status of an animal is well recognized as having an important influence on drug metabolism, disposition and toxicity. The lack of various nutrients may affect drug metabolism, though not always causing a depression of metabolic activity. Lack of protein has been particularly well studied in this respect, and shows a marked influence on drug metabolism. Thus, rats fed on low-protein diets show a marked loss of microsomal enzyme activity *in vitro*, there being a greater than twofold difference from those animals fed a 20% protein diet. The effect occurs within 24 hours on a low protein diet (5%) and reaches a minimum level after four days. The decline in activity is accompanied by a decline in the level of liver microsomal protein. Both cytochrome P-450 content and cytochrome P-450 reductase activity are reduced by a 5% protein diet.

Measurements *in vivo*, such as barbiturate sleeping times, are in agreement with these findings, sleeping times being longer in protein-deficient animals. Toxicity may also be influenced by such factors as a low-protein diet. For example, the hepatotoxicity of carbon tetrachloride is markedly less in protein-deficient rats than in normal animals, and this correlates with the reduced ability to metabolize the hepatotoxin in the protein-deficient animals. However, the reverse is the case with the hepatotoxicity of paracetamol, which is increased after a low-protein diet. This may be due to the reduced levels of glutathione in rats fed low-protein diets, which offsets the reduced amount of cytochrome P-450 caused by protein deficiency.

The carcinogenicity of aflatoxin is reduced by protein deficiency, presumably because of reduced metabolic activation to the epoxide intermediate which may be the ultimate carcinogen which binds to DNA (figure 5.17). The nutritional status of an animal may affect the disposition of a foreign compound *in vivo* as well as the metabolism. Many drugs are protein-bound in the plasma, and alteration of the extent of binding for compounds extensively bound may have important toxicological implications. Thus, the decreased plasma levels of albumin after low-protein diets, such as occur in the human deficiency disease Kwashiorkor, might lead to significantly increased plasma levels of the free drug and therefore the possibility of increased toxicity.

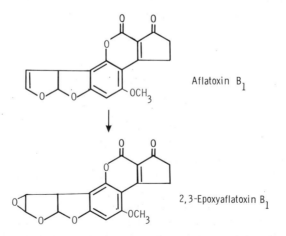

Aflatoxin B$_1$

2,3-Epoxyaflatoxin B$_1$

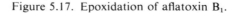

Figure 5.17. Epoxidation of aflatoxin B$_1$.

Age effects

It is well known that the drug-metabolizing capacity and various other metabolic and physiological functions in man and other animals are influenced by age. Furthermore, sensitivity to the toxic and pharmacological effects of drugs and other foreign compounds is often greater in young and geriatric animals. As might be expected, at the extremes of age, drug-metabolizing activity is often impaired, plasma-protein binding capacity is altered and the clearance of foreign compounds from the body may be less efficient. These differences generally lead to exposure to a higher level of unchanged drug for longer periods in the young and geriatric animals than in adults, with all the implications for toxicity that this has. The case of the foetus is rather special, because of the influence of the maternal organism, and will therefore be considered separately at the end of this section.

Although the toxicological significance has yet to be studied, age-related differences in the absorption of foreign compounds are demonstrable. Neonatal and geriatric human subjects have low gastric acidity, and consequently the absorption of some compounds, such as penicillin, may be enhanced. Intestinal motility may also be influenced by age, with various effects on the absorption of foreign compounds dependent upon the site of such absorption. The absence of gut flora in the neonate may have as yet unknown influences on the disposition of foreign compounds in the gastrointestinal tract.

Once absorbed, foreign compounds may react with plasma proteins and distribute into various body compartments. Although in human neonates plasma albumin concentration is at the adult level at birth, in elderly subjects it may be reduced by 20%, which could result in a reduction in plasma binding capacity.

Total body water, particularly extracellular water, has been found to be greater in neonates than in adults and to decrease with age. The distribution of water-soluble drugs could clearly be influenced by this, lower plasma levels being one possible result. Both glomerular filtration and renal tubular secretion are lower in neonates and geriatrics, and human infants achieve adult levels only by six months to one year of age. The consequences of this are reduced excretion, and hence reduced body clearance of foreign compounds. Consequently, toxicity may be increased by prolongation of exposure or accumulation if chronic dosing is involved.

Many drug-metabolizing enzyme systems show marked changes around the time of birth, being generally reduced in the foetus and neonate. In some cases, adult activity may be achieved within a few days, whereas for some enzymes, such as cytochrome P-450, several weeks may be necessary to obtain optimum levels.

Table 5.14. Effect of age on metabolism and duration of action of hexobarbital.

Age (days)	Percent hexobarbital metabolized *in vitro*† in 1 h (guinea-pigs)	Percent hexobarbital metabolized *in vivo* in 3 h (mice)	Sleeping time in mice (min)		
			(10 mg/kg)	(50 mg/kg)	(100 mg/kg)
1	0	0	> 360	Died	Died
7	2·5–3·5	11–24	107 ± 26	243 ± 30	> 360
21	13–21	21–33	27 ± 11	64 ± 17	94 ± 27
Adult	28–39		< 5	17 ± 5	47 ± 11

† Guinea-pig liver microsomes.
Data of Jondorf *et al.* (1958) *Biochem. Pharmac.*, **1**, 352.

When the parent compound is responsible for the pharmacological or toxicological effect, reduced metabolic activity may lead to prolonged and exaggerated responses. For example, in mice there is very little oxidation of the side-chain of hexobarbital, and the sleeping time is excessively prolonged (by 70 times), as shown in table 5.14. Doses giving sleeping times of less than one hour in adult mice are fatally toxic to neonates. This activity correlates with the inability to metabolize the drug.

The converse is true of drugs requiring metabolic activation for toxicity. For example, paracetamol is less hepatotoxic to newborn than to adult mice, as less is metabolically activated in the neonate. This is due to the lower levels of cytochrome P-450 in neonatal liver (figure 5.18). Also involved in this is the hepatic level of glutathione, which is required for detoxication. Although levels of this tripeptide are reduced at birth, development is sufficiently in advance of cytochrome P-450 levels to ensure adequate detoxication (figure 5.18). The same effect has been observed with the hepatotoxin bromobenzene. (For further details of paracetamol and bromobenzene see Chapter 7.) Other enzyme activities at low or unmeasurable levels *in vitro* in the neonate are the *N*-demethylation of methyl aminoantipyrine, the *o*-de-ethylation of phenacetin (figure 5.13), the deamination of amphetamine (figure 4.25), the aromatic hydroxylation of acetanilide, the oxidation of sulphur in chlorpromazine and the reduction of *p*-nitrobenzoic acid. For instance, studies of acetanilide metabolism in human infants *in vivo* support the *in vitro* data from experimental animals.

Conjugating enzymes are also of lower activity in young animals and in

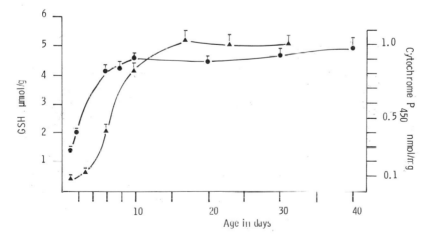

Figure 5.18. Development of hepatic reduced glutathione and cytochrome P-450 levels with age in mice. Glutathione (●), cytochrome P-450 (▲). Data of Hart & Timbrell (1979) *Biochem. Pharmac.*, **28**, 3015.

human infants. For example, the low level of glucuronyl transferase which may occur in human babies is responsible for the condition of neonatal jaundice. This is due to high levels of unconjugated bilirubin in the plasma, and may be exacerbated by the administration of drugs which displace bilirubin from its binding sites on plasma proteins.

A most tragic example of enhanced toxicity due to lowered glucuronyl transferase activity is that of chloramphenicol toxicity in human infants. This drug is normally largely detoxified and excreted as a glucuronide conjugate, to the extent of about 90% in human adults. The lowered activity of glucuronyl transferase in human neonates results in high plasma levels of unchanged chloramphenicol and severe cyanosis with sometimes a fatal outcome. This toxic effect may also reflect, in part, reduced renal clearance of the drug in the neonate.

Drug-metabolizing capacity in elderly subjects has been less well studied, but the indications are that it is less than in younger adults. One might therefore predict similar pharmacological and toxicological consequences.

The situation with regard to the foetus is a rather special case. Although many of the same comments apply to the foetus as to neonatal animals, the relationship with the maternal circulation exerts a modifying effect. Thus, clearance of compounds from foetal plasma may be more efficient, although if polar compounds are produced in the foetal liver, these may be unable to leave the embryo because they are unable to cross the placenta. Alternatively, drugs ingested by the mother may be metabolized maternally and then be unable to cross the placenta. However, most drugs, particularly on chronic administration, attain the same steady-state levels in the foetal as in the maternal plasma, unless metabolism and/or excretion by the foetus is significant. The foetal kidney, however, excretes certain compounds into the allantoic fluid. Plasma-protein binding capacity is less in the foetus due to lower levels of albumin. The ability of the foetus to metabolize foreign compounds is generally less than that of the adult animal, as it is with the neonate. However, this may depend on the metabolic pathway and enzyme system involved.

Cytochrome P-450 shows negligible activity in the foetus until birth, although activity is measurable in embryonic tissue. This is the case in most mammals, except man, where the foetus six weeks after gestation shows measurable cytochrome P-450 activity which is between 20% and 40% of adult values by mid-term, this level being maintained until birth.

Glucoronyl-transferase activity has been shown to be low in the foetus, using substrates such as *p*-nitrophenol and 1-naphthol (figures 4.8 and 4.42). Diazepam is metabolized to *N*-demethyldiazepam, which is conjugated with glucuronic acid in adults and children; however, no glucuronide is detectable in premature infants. It is clear that if cytochrome P-450 activity is present in the foetus but conjugating ability is impaired, toxic metabolites rather than stable, less toxic conjugates could accumulate.

The activity of cytosolic enzymes such as the glutathione transferases is also lower in the foetus, being only 5–10 % of the adult value in rabbits and guinea-pigs. The glutathione content of foetal mouse liver was found to be approximately 10 % of that of the adult, but studies indicate that the mouse foetus is still protected from the hepatotoxic effects of compounds such as paracetamol by this level of glutathione.

It is therefore apparent that the foetus may not always be at greater risk from the toxic effects of foreign compounds than the neonate. Its susceptibility depends very much on the particular compound. The human neonate, however, may be unusual in having a comparatively high level of microsomal enzyme activity, which may have important toxicological consequences for the foetus exposed to compounds metabolized by such enzymes to more toxic products. The rapidity of clearance of the compound from the maternal circulation is of paramount importance to the foetal toxicity of a foreign compound. Teratogenicity is a special case of foetal toxicity in its dependence on the stage of development, and will be considered in a later chapter.

Effects of pathological conditions

The influence of disease in the disposition of foreign compounds is potentially an important factor in the toxicity of such compounds. Drugs are generally given to humans suffering from one of a variety of diseases, whereas most of the information on the disposition and toxicity of these drugs arises from studies in normal experimental animals and healthy human volunteers. Relatively little is known of the influence of pathological changes on toxicity.

The absorption of foreign compounds from the gastrointestinal tract may be altered in certain malabsorption syndromes, and may be increased after subcutaneous or intramuscular injection if vasodilation accompanies the particular disease. The disposition of foreign compounds, once absorbed, can be influenced by changes in plasma proteins, which are sometimes reduced in certain disease states. Consequently, for foreign compounds which are highly protein-bound, the plasma concentration of the free compound may be significantly increased in such circumstances. This may alter renal excretion, increasing it in some cases, but could also increase the toxicity of a drug with a narrow therapeutic ratio if the compound dissociated from the protein was responsible for the toxicity. Thus, thiopental anaesthesia is prolonged when plasma albumin is reduced by chronic liver disease, and more unbound diphenylhydantoin and sulphonamides result from changes in plasma proteins in chronic liver disease.

The influence of liver disease and damage itself on drug disposition is not at present clear but must also be considered. Although such damage results in reduced metabolism in experimental animals, this is not always the case in humans.

It is possible that the severity of liver damage and hence dysfunction is the major factor. Although the half-life of isoniazid was found to be prolonged in patients with liver disease, this was not a major effect compared with the effect of the acetylator phenotype.

Mild to moderate hepatitis in man was not found to influence hepatic cytochrome P-450 content or activity, content being reduced by 50% in severe hepatitis and cirrhosis. Acute hepatic necrosis caused by the administration of hepatotoxins results in decreased metabolism of barbiturates, diphenylhydantoin and antipyrine, giving an approximate doubling of the plasma half-life. Extra-hepatic drug metabolism may also be influenced by liver disease, for example, the activity of the plasma esterase involved in succinylcholine and procaine hydrolysis is reduced in this pathological condition.

The impaired formation of glucuronic acid and sulphate conjugates is known to occur in several types of liver disease, such as cirrhosis, hepatitis and obstructive jaundice. Decreased ability to form glucuronides may also occur in Gilbert's disease and the Crigler–Najjer syndrome. In these genetic disorders, glucuronyl transferase is reduced and consequently bilirubin conjugation may be affected when drugs which are also conjugated with glucuronic acid are administered.

Renal disease is another important factor, particularly if renal excretion is the major route of elimination for the pharmacologically or toxicologically active compound. This may be particularly important with drugs showing a low therapeutic ratio, such as digoxin and the aminoglycoside antibiotics. As already mentioned, plasma protein binding may be affected in renal disease, such binding being reduced particularly with regard to organic acids. Increased toxicity of drugs undergoing significant metabolism, such as chloramphenicol, has been found in uraemic patients. The half-lives of a number of drugs are prolonged in renal failure, although this effect is variable and by no means the general rule, different drugs being differently affected. Hepatic metabolism may also be influenced by renal failure, although there is little clear data on this, much more data being required in the area of pathological effects on the disposition and toxicity of foreign compounds.

Tissue and organ specificity

The disposition or localization and in some cases metabolism of foreign compounds may be dependent upon the characteristics of a particular tissue or organ which may in turn affect the toxicity. There are many examples of organotropy in toxicology, but the mechanisms underlying such organ-specific toxic effects are often unknown.

It is clear that a foreign compound which is chemically similar to, or at least has certain structural similarities with, an endogenous compound may become localized in a particular tissue(s). An example of this is 6-hydroxy-dopamine, a single dose of which is selectively toxic to sympathetic nerve endings. Because of its similarity with noradrenaline, 6-hydroxydopamine is distributed specifically to the sympathetic nerve endings. There it is oxidized to a quinone (figure 7.17), which binds covalently to the nerve endings and permanently inactivates them. In other cases, however, the mechanism of specificity is less clear. Certain carcinogens show organ or tissue specificity, such as *trans*-4-dimethylaminostilbene, which causes earduct tumours after repeated administration, or hydrazine, which causes lung tumours (figure 5.19). This may reflect the ability of the tissue to carry out repair of damaged macromolecules, such as DNA. Thus, if DNA repair is poor in a particular tissue, such as nervous tissue, that tissue may be particularly susceptible to certain carcinogens. The carcinogen diethylstilboestrol induces tumours in those female organs particularly exposed to oestrogens, namely the mammary glands, uterus and vagina (figure 6.13). In male hamsters, however, this compound causes kidney tumours.

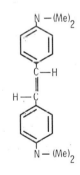

4-Dimethylaminostilbene

NH_2NH_2

Hydrazine

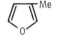

3-Methylfuran

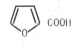

2-Furoic Acid

Figure 5.19. Structure of 4-dimethylaminostilbene, hydrazine, 2-methylfuran and 2-furoic acid.

Although certain organs are prime targets for toxic effects because of their anatomical position and function, such as the gut, liver and kidney, they may not necessarily be the most susceptible. Such organs may have a particular ability to cope with a toxic insult, and this has been termed *reserve functional capacity*. Examples of organ-specific toxicity are the lung toxicity of the natural furan ipomeanol (figure 7.13), 3-methylfuran (figure 5.19), the herbicide paraquat (figure 3.7) and the kidney toxicity of chloroform, 2-furoic acid (figure 5.19) and *p*-aminophenol (figure 5.4). However, some of these compounds, such as 3-methylfuran and paraquat, are rarely, if ever, hepatotoxic, even after oral administration. The lung toxin ipomeanol is considered in greater detail in the final chapter (see page 200).

The phospholipidoses caused by certain amphiphilic drugs typified by chlorphentermine (figure 2.3) tend to be organ- and tissue-specific, occurring particularly in the lungs and adrenals. This correlates with the accumulation of the drug, which is localized in the fatty tissue, particularly that associated with the adrenals and lungs (pages 12–13).

Dose

It is clear from Chapter 2 that the dose of a toxic compound is a major factor in its toxicity. This may be a simple relationship resulting from the increasing concentration of toxin at its site of action, with a proportional increase in response with increasing dose. However, the size of the dose may also influence the disposition or metabolism of the compound.

Thus, a large dose may be ineffectively distributed and remain at the site of administration as a depot. A large dose of a compound given orally, for instance, may not be all absorbed, depending on the rates of absorption and transit time within the gut. Saturable active absorption processes would be particularly prone to dose effects, which could result in unexpected dose–response relationships.

Once a toxic compound has been absorbed, the disposition of it *in vivo* may also be affected by the dose. Thus, saturation of plasma-protein binding sites may lead to a significant rise in the plasma concentration of free compound, with possible toxic effects. This, of course, depends on the fraction of the compound that is bound, and is only of significance with highly protein-bound substances. The result of this is a disproportionate rise in toxicity for a small increase in dose.

Saturation of the processes involved in the elimination of a foreign compound from the plasma, such as metabolism and excretion, may also have toxicological consequences. Thus, ethanol exhibits zero-order elimination kinetics at readily attainable plasma concentrations, because the metabolism is readily saturated. Therefore, once these plasma concentrations have been attained, the rate of elimination from the plasma is constant. Increasing the dosage of ethanol leads to accumulation and the well known toxic effects.

The biliary excretion of furosemide is also an active process and saturable, and after high doses of furosemide there is a disproportionate increase in the plasma level of the drug. This appears to be responsible for the toxic dose threshold, above which hepatic necrosis ensues (figures 3.19 and 3.20, page 45).

The metabolism of toxic compounds may also be influenced by dose, with possible toxicological consequences. Saturation of metabolic routes may increase toxicity if the parent compound is more toxic than its metabolites, or if minor but toxic routes become more important. Conversely, toxicity may not increase proportionately with dose if the pathway responsible becomes saturated. For example, paracetamol hepatotoxicity is dose-dependent but only above a threshold dose. This threshold is the result of saturation of the glutathione conjugation pathway. Another example is isoniazid hepatotoxicity, which results from an acetylated metabolite. Giving large doses of isoniazid to experimental animals does not cause hepatic necrosis, whereas giving several smaller doses does, probably because acetylation is saturated at high doses and the drug is metabolized by other routes. Both these examples are discussed in greater detail in the final chapter.

Enzyme induction and inhibition

Compounds which induce or inhibit the activity of the enzymes involved in the metabolism of foreign compounds may be very important factors in the toxicity of such compounds. The number of inhibitors, and particularly the number of inducing agents, is large and includes drugs, environmental pollutants, natural products and pesticides. There are several enzyme systems which may be affected in a variety of tissues, and the effects are generally common to more than one species.

Chronic exposure to some inducing agents or inhibitors, for instance, may be a major factor in the development of a toxic response to another compound, which may not always be recognized. Thus, our diet may be one such factor, either because of the natural products it contains, the pesticides it may be contaminated with, or the food additives it is supplied with.

Enzyme induction

The induction of microsomal enzymes has been demonstrated in many different species, including man, and in several different tissues from these species. Induction may require the repeated administration of the compound or chronic exposure to it. Although the most well known and studied microsomal enzyme system stimulated by other compounds is the cytochrome P-450 mono-oxygenase system, other enzymes also may be induced. Thus, microsomal enzyme-catalysed reduction, glucuronyl transferase, UDP-glucose dehydrogenase, glutathione transferases and esterases, as well as some of the enzymes involved in steroid metabolism, can all be induced by microsomal enzyme inducers.

The major types of microsomal enzyme inducer are the barbiturates, typified by phenobarbital, and the polycyclic hydrocarbons, of which 3-methylcholanthrene is the best known. However, these two inducers produce different effects. Although the two compounds induce the microsomal mono-oxygenase system, each induces a different form of the cytochrome P-450 with different spectral properties. Phenobarbital causes a proliferation of the smooth endoplasmic reticulum, whereas 3-methylcholanthrene does not. It seems that the induction caused by phenobarbital is fairly general, whereas that of 3-methylcholanthrene is more specific. As well as increasing the amount of cytochrome P-450, phenobarbital also increases NADPH cytochrome P-450 reductase and RNA synthesis.

It seems that induction is basically a cellular phenomenon occurring within the microsomes. Thus, in isolated cells, such as hamster foetal cells growing in culture, induction of microsomal enzymes such as benzo[a]pyrene hydroxylase occurs if an inducer such as benzo[a]anthracene is included in the medium. Induction is accompanied by an increase in messenger RNA synthesis and protein synthesis, and can be blocked by treatment with actinomycin D, an mRNA synthesis inhibitor, and other inhibitors such as cycloheximide and puromycin. The data suggests that an increase in *de novo* synthesis of enzyme protein takes place. This may be the result of a genetic interaction, possibly combination with a repressor gene to allow de-repression of the operator gene and hence the synthesis of mRNA (see Chapter 6, page 162).

Conney has summarized the possible interactions. Inducers may interact with (a) DNA to stimulate DNA-directed synthesis of mRNA; (b) with repressors or other regulators of gene function; (c) with the endoplasmic reticulum to enhance translation of mRNA on the ribosomes; and (d) with mono-oxygenases, to reduce activity and hence allow an endogenous inducing agent to accumulate.

It is of particular interest that many inducing agents are also inhibitors of the microsomal enzymes when given as a single dose. The latter observation and the fact that a very wide variety of compounds are inducers is supportive of the concept of an endogenous derepressor which accumulates on inhibition of cytochrome P-450. Inducers are known to increase δ-aminolaevulinate synthetase activity, which is the rate-limiting enzyme of haem synthesis, with a consequent increase in the synthesis of haem.

Inducers may cause changes other than those in the microsomal enzymes. Phenobarbital induction, for instance, also leads to an increase in liver blood flow and biliary flow. Interference with steroid metabolism may occur and may have physiological complications. For example, treatment with the drug rifampicin, an antitubercular drug administered chronically, and a well known inducing agent, may lead to contraceptive steroids becoming ineffective.

In terms of toxicity, enzyme induction may either increase or decrease the toxic effects of a particular compound, depending on the basis for that toxicity. Different inducers also influence toxicity differently. For instance, with the inducers DDT, 3MC and chlordane, only treatment with chlordane protects against parathion toxicity. Phenobarbital induction increases the toxicity of phosphorothionate insecticides, but reduces that of other organophosphate insecticides. The pharmacological activity of codeine is increased by induction, as this increases demethylation to morphine. The toxicity of cyclophosphamide is increased by induction with the inducer chlordane.

Therefore, prediction of the toxicological effects of enzyme inducers requires some prior knowledge of the metabolism and toxicity. Although induction may increase the activity of a toxic pathway, it may also increase that of non-toxic pathways with a net decrease in toxicity. Specific examples of this are discussed in more detail in the final chapter.

There are now many examples of environmental enzyme-inducing agents, the effects of some of which have been studied in human subjects. For instance, the influence of dietary polycyclic hydrocarbons derived from steak grilled over charcoal, and the effect of cigarette smoking on drug metabolism and disposition has been well studied in human subjects. Charcoal-grilled meat contains benzo[a]pyrene and human subjects fed various diets and given the drug phenacetin were found to have significantly lower plasma levels of the drug after a diet containing beef cooked over charcoal. This was due to the increased de-ethylation of phenacetin to paracetamol, which is a microsomal enzyme-mediated pathway (figure 5.13). Similar results were obtained in subjects who smoked cigarettes. These results show that a large difference in the metabolism of a drug may occur because of enzyme induction. The plasma level of phenacetin was reduced to 20–25% of normal levels by the charcoal-grilled steak diet, although there was no difference in half-life, as phenacetin undergoes a significant first-pass effect. Such an effect could have important toxicological consequences, which would depend on whether the metabolite was more or less toxic than the parent compound, whether the rate of production was an important factor and whether the proportions of metabolites were affected.

Studies in laboratory animals have shown that the toxicity of foreign compounds can be markedly increased by the induction of the microsomal enzymes, and the data available from humans suggests that the same may be true in man. Of particular importance is the relationship with long-term

E

toxic effects such as carcinogenesis, where it is difficult to know which of a number of environmental factors is important in the development of toxicity.

Microsomal enzymes which are involved in conjugation reactions, such as glucuronyl transferase and epoxide hydratase, may also be induced. Induction of these enzymes may lead to a decrease in toxicity, as for example in paracetamol andb romobenzene hepatotoxicity, discussed in more detail in Chapter 7.

Genetics of induction

Studies in mice and rats have revealed that certain strains are non-responsive to the effects of inducing agents. Thus, the inducibility of aryl hydrocarbon hydroxylase by polycyclic hydrocarbons can be shown to be strain-dependent in mice, and evidence also suggests a genetic basis in man.

The studies in mice have indicated that the inducibility of this microsomal enzyme may be dependent on a single dominant gene locus, the Ah locus. It may be that the cytosolic receptor for the inducing agent is the product of a single gene, and that differences in this gene are responsible for the differences in inducibility.

Enzyme inhibition

In contrast to enzyme induction, inhibition generally only requires a single dose of inhibitor rather than repeated doses. Although environmentally it may be of less consequence than induction, in the case of drug interactions it is probably of greater importance. There are few microsomal enzyme inhibitors which have been well studied. However, apart from the enzymes located in the microsomes, there are a number of enzymes involved in drug metabolism the inhibition of which may have toxicological consequences.

One of the best known and studied microsomal enzyme inhibitors is SKF 525A. This compound inhibits many but not all microsomal enzyme reactions, including glucuronyl transferase in some cases, and also the hydrolysis of procaine, a non-microsomal enzyme-mediated reaction. Its mechanism of action is unclear, seeming to involve competitive inhibition in some cases but non-competitive inhibition in others. There is no doubt, however, that it binds to cytochrome P-450 and inhibits microsomal enzymes both *in vivo* and *in vitro*.

Another widely used microsomal enzyme inhibitor is piperonyl butoxide, a member of the methylenedioxyphenyl insecticide synergists. These compounds probably function as alternative substrates and are active *in vivo* but less so *in vitro*. Piperonyl butoxide, however, may also influence synthesis of cytochrome P-450 by its action on δ-aminolaevulinate synthetase, the rate-limiting step of haem biosynthesis. Its action as an insecticide synergist is dependent on its being administered at the same time. The insect, unable to metabolize the synergist, shows increased toxicity to the insecticide. For instance, the carbamate insecticide carbaryl (figure 4.42) is mixed with 2,3-methylenedioxynaphthalene, a synergist. Toxicity of the mixture to house flies was seen at 5 µg/g, whereas no toxicity was observed in mice after 750 mg/kg. This is due to the ability of the mouse to metabolize the synergist and hence allow microsomal metabolism of the insecticide.

A clinically important example of microsomal enzyme inhibition is that caused by the drug isoniazid. This may have serious consequences, for example when isoniazid is administered with diphenylhydantoin, an anti-epileptic drug. Termination of the pharmacological activity of diphenyl-hydantoin depends on microsomal metabolism (figure 7.21) which may be inhibited by isoniazid when they are administered together. The consequence of this is the appearance of toxic effects after therapeutic doses of both drugs are taken, and the plasma half-life of diphenylhydantoin is significantly increased (page 210).

Inhibitors of other enzymes may also be important in toxicology. For instance, salicylamide inhibits both the glucuronidation and sulphation of paracetamol and thereby increases its toxicity, as will be explained in greater detail in Chapter 7.

Certain enzyme inhibitors such as allopurinol and disulphiram are used clinically. Allopurinol blocks xanthine oxidase *in vivo*, and consequently inhibits the metabolism of compounds such as 6-mercaptopurine (figure 4.17), thereby increasing its anticancer efficacy. Chronic treatment with allopurinol inhibits the metabolism of other compounds such as bis-hydroxycoumarin, increasing the half-life of this drug threefold.

Disulphiram inhibits aldehyde dehydrogenase *in vivo*, and is used to treat alcoholism, as it allows acetaldehyde to accumulate after alcohol ingestion, with consequent toxic effects. The inhibition is irreversible, non-competitive with acetaldehyde and has a half-life of about 24 hours. Other enzymes are also inhibited by disulphiram, including microsomal mono-oxygenases. Chronic disulphiram treatment depresses cytochrome P-450 levels and hence decreases aniline hydroxylase and ethylmorphine *N*-demethylase.

Administration of diphenylhydantoin after disulphiram therapy may lead to toxicity due to the impaired metabolism of diphenylhydantoin in the same way as was described for the interaction with isoniazid (see above). The toxicity of 1,2-dimethylhydrazine, a colon carcinogen, was found to be inhibited by disulphiram treatment. 1,2-Dimethylhydrazine is metabolized to azomethane, which undergoes *N*-oxidation to azoxymethane (figure 5.20). This oxidation step, essential for the carcinogenicity of 1,2-dimethylhydrazine, is inhibited by disulphiram. Exposure to esterase and amidase inhibitors may have important toxicological consequences, as they are often long-acting. Many insecticides are inhibitors of this type, and humans, such as agricultural workers, and

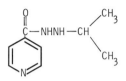

Figure 5.20. Metabolism of 1,2-dimethylhydrazine.

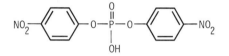

Iproniazid

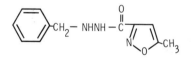

bis-*p*-Nitrophenyl phosphate

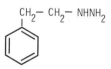

Isocarboxazid

CH₂— CH₂— NHNH₂

Phenelzine

Figure 5.21. Structures of the enzyme inhibitors bis-*p*-nitrophenyl phosphate (BNPP), iproniazid, phenelzine and isocarboxazid.

animals which are exposed to them, acutely or chronically, could be at risk. Many such insecticides are organophosphate, carbamate or phosphoro-thionate derivatives. They act as substrates for the esterases and amidases but inactivate the enzyme by binding irreversibly to the active site or binding for prolonged periods. The exact mechanism of this inhibition is discussed in more detail in Chapter 7.

Bis-*p*-nitrophenylphosphate is an acylamidase inhibitor of the organophosphate type (figure 5.21). It has been used as an experimental tool to investigate the toxicity of certain acylamides and hydrazides, such as phenacetin and acetylisoniazid respectively (figures 5.13 and 4.41). The drug phenacetin may cause methaemoglobinaemia (see page 104), which results from the oxidation of haemoglobin, in both experimental animals and man. This is thought to be due to the metabolite 2-hydroxyphenetidine (figure 5.13), a product of hydroxylation and deacetylation. This deacetylation is blocked by bis-*p*-nitrophenylphosphate and therefore the methaemoglobin formation *in vivo* from phenacetin in experimental animals is also blocked by the amidase inhibitor. Esterase and amidase inhibition may have important toxicological effects by interfering with normal metabolic processes such as the hydrolysis of acetylcholine, as well as by inhibiting the biotransformation of other compounds and thereby influencing their toxicity.

The mitochondrial enzyme, monoamine oxidase, may be inhibited by certain foreign compounds such as the antidepressant drugs iproniazid, phenelzine and isocarboxazid, which are all substituted hydrazine derivatives (figure 5.21). The hydrazine monoamine oxidase inhibitors are thought to act as substrates for the enzyme, but once bound irreversibly they block the active site. Iproniazid will completely inhibit monoamine oxidase for 24 hours and normal activity does not return for five days. Inhibition of monoamine oxidase may be important if the organism is exposed to amines normally metabolized by oxidative deamination, and a particular example of this is exposure to amines such as tyramine or drugs of the phenylethylamine group. Ingestion of tyramine in foodstuffs such as cheese can lead to severe hypertensive effects in patients taking monoamine oxidase inhibitors. The inhibited enzyme is unable to metabolize amines normally, with a consequent potentiation of the cardiovascular effects of the tyramine.

Bibliography

General

DOULL, J. (1980) Factors influencing toxicology. In *Cassaret and Doull's Toxicology, The Basic Science of Poisons*, edited by J. Doull, C. D. Klaassen and M. O. Amdur (New York: Macmillan).

GOLDSTEIN, A., ARONOW, L. & KALMAN, S. M. (1974) Drug metabolism. *Principles of Drug Action: The Basis of Pharmacology* (New York: John Wiley).

HODGSON, E. & GUTHRIE, F. E. (editors) (1980) *Introduction to Biochemical Toxicology*, Chapters 6, 7 and 8 (New York: Elsevier-North Holland).
PARKE, D. V. (1968) *The Biochemistry of Foreign Compounds*, Chapter 6 (Oxford: Pergamon).

Species, strain and sex effects

ADAMSON, R. H. & DAVIES, D. S. (1973) Comparative aspects of absorption, distribution, metabolism and excretion of drugs. In *International Encyclopaedia of Pharmacology and Therapeutics*, Section 85, Chapter 9 (Oxford: Pergamon).
HATHWAY, D. E., BROWN, S. S., CHASSEAUD, L. F. & HUTSON, D. H. (reporters) (1970–1981) *Foreign Compound Metabolism in Mammals*, Vols. 1–6 (London: The Chemical Society). (This series contains chapters on species, strain and sex differences in metabolism.)
HUCKER, H. B. (1970) Species differences in drug metabolism. *Ann. Rev. Pharmac.*, **10,** 99.
PARKE, D. V. (1968) *The Biochemistry of Foreign Compounds*, Chapter 7 (Oxford: Pergamon).
SMITH, R. L. (1970) Species differences in the biliary excretion of drugs. In *Problems of Species Difference and Statistics in Toxicology, Proc. Eur. Soc. Study Drug Tox.*, Vol. XI, edited by S. B. Baker, J. Tripod and J. Jacob.
WILLIAMS, R. T. (1974) Interspecies variations in the metabolism of xenobiotics. *Biochem. Soc. Trans.*, **2,** 359.

Genetic factors

BOOBIS, A. R. (1979) Genetic factors affecting side effects of drugs. In *Drug Toxicity*, edited by J. W. Gorrod (London: Taylor & Francis).
IDLE, J. R. & SMITH, R. L. (1979) Polymorphisms of oxidation at carbon centers of drugs and their clinical significance. *Drug. Metab. Rev.*, **9,** 301.
NEBERT, D. W. & FELTON, J. S. (1976) Importance of genetic factors influencing the metabolism of foreign compounds. *Fed. Proc.*, **35,** 1133.
VESELL, E. S. (1975) Genetically determined variations in drug disposition and response in man. In *Handbook of Experimental Pharmacology*, Vol. 28, Part 3, *Concepts in Biochemical Pharmacology*, edited by J. R. Gillette and J. R. Mitchell (Berlin: Springer Verlag).
WEBER, W. W., DRUMMOND, G., MICELI, J. N. & SZABADI, R. (1975) Genetic control and isozymic composition of drug acetylating enzymes. In *Isozymes*, edited by C. L. Market (New York: Academic Press).

Diet

ANGELI-GREAVES, M. & MCLEAN, A. E. M. (1979) The effect of diet on the toxicity of drugs. In *Drug Toxicity*, edited by J. W. Gorrod (London: Taylor & Francis).

CAMBELL, T. C., HAYES, J. R., MERRILL, A. H., MASO, M. & GOETCHIUS, M. (1979) The influence of dietary factors on drug metabolism in animals. *Drug Metab. Rev.*, **9**, 173.

DOLLERY, C. T., FRASER, H. S., MUCKLOW, J. C. & BULPITT, C. J. (1979) Contribution of environmental factors to variability in human drug metabolism. *Drug Metab. Rev.*, **9**, 207.

Age

GILLETTE, J. R. & STRIPP, B. (1975) Pre- and postnatal enzyme capacity for drug metabolite production. *Fed. Proc.*, **34**, 172.

NEIMS, A. H., WARNER, M., LOUGHNAN, P. M. & ARANDA, J. V. (1976) Developmental aspects of the hepatic cytochrome P 450 mono-oxygenase system. *Ann. Rev. Pharmac. Toxicol.*, **16**, 427.

SCHMUCKER, D. L. (1979) Age-related changes in drug disposition. *Pharmac. Rev.*, **30**, 445.

Pathological conditions

PRESCOTT, L. F. (1975) Pathological and physiological factors affecting drug absorption, distribution, elimination and response in man. In *Handbook of Experimental Pharmacology*, Vol. 28, Part 3, *Concepts in Biochemical Pharmacology*, edited by J. R. Gillette and J. R. Mitchell (Berlin: Springer Verlag).

Tissue and organ specificity

CHAMBERS, P. L. & GUNSEL, P. (editors) (1979) Mechanism of toxic action on some target organs. *Archs Toxicol.*, Suppl. 2.

GRAM, T. E. (editor) (1980) *Extrahepatic Metabolism of Drugs and Other Foreign Compounds* (Jamaica, New York: Spectrum Publications).

Enzyme induction

ALVARES, A. P., PANTUCK, E. J., ANDERSON, K. E., KAPPAS, A. & CONNEY, A. H. (1979) Regulation of drug metabolism in man by environmental factors. *Drug Metab. Rev.*, **9**, 185.

CONNEY, A. H. (1967) Pharmacological implications of microsomal enzyme induction. *Pharmac. Rev.*, **19**, 317.

SNYDER, R. & REMMER, H. (1979) Classes of hepatic microsomal mixed function oxidase inducers. *Pharmac. Ther.*, **7**, 203.

Enzyme inhibition

ANDERS, M. W. (1971) Enhancement and inhibition of drug metabolism. *Ann. Rev. Pharmac.*, **11**, 37.

Chapter 6

Toxic responses to foreign compounds

Introduction

There are many ways in which an organism may respond to a toxic compound, and the type of response depends upon numerous factors. Although many of the toxic effects of foreign compounds have a biochemical basis, the expression of the effects may be very different. Thus, the development of tumours may be one result of an attack on nucleic acids, another might be the birth of an abnormal offspring. The interaction of a toxic compound with normal metabolic processes may cause a physiological response such as muscle paralysis, or a fall in blood pressure, or it may cause a tissue lesion in one organ. The covalent interaction between a toxic foreign compound and a normal body protein may in some circumstances cause an immunological response, in others a tissue lesion.

Thus, although all these toxic responses may have a biochemical basis, they have been categorized according to the manifestation of the toxic effect.

Chemical carcinogenesis

Introduction

Study of the induction of cancer by chemicals has become a large, highly complex and rapidly changing field of scientific research. The pathological and biochemical changes which take place have been and continue to be studied in great detail. Consequently, it is beyond the scope of this book to attempt more than a brief overview of this particular area of toxicology. However, three specific carcinogens are considered in more detail in Chapter 7.

It is now generally accepted that the vast majority of human cancers are caused by environmental agents, mainly the many and various foreign chemicals to which we are exposed, and to a lesser extent radiation and viruses. The number of known chemical carcinogens is now large, and they exhibit a diverse range of chemical structures (figure 6.1).

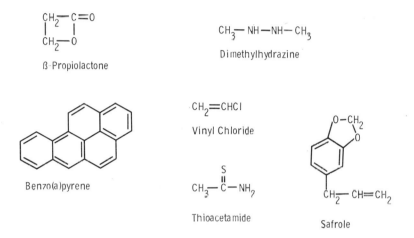

Figure 6.1. Structures of various carcinogens

The induction of cancer is usually an irreversible, often life-threatening change, and consequently the study and understanding of chemical carcinogenesis is of major importance. Although environmental chemicals may be a major factor, other factors such as genetic predisposition must also be taken into account, although their role is as yet unclear.

The cancerous cell is a somatic cell indulging in unrestrained, malignant proliferation. The trait is heritable, as tumour cells give rise to more tumour cells. The induction of cancer involves at least two events, first the initiation stage and then a promotional stage. Thus the interaction of the carcinogen with a cell produces, in most cases, an irreversible change, which may then be promoted by further factors into the development of a tumour. This promotional step may involve proliferation of cells and hence replication of DNA. Croton oil and its constituent phorbol esters are well known promoters, but their specific mode of action is still unclear.

The induction of a tumour by a chemical carcinogen therefore involves a direct or indirect reaction with informational macromolecules such as nucleic acids, which leads to the changes in growth control characteristic of malignant transformations. There may be many cellular targets for such interactions with the ultimate carcinogen, and the critical targets are not yet clearly defined. Although interactions with nucleic acids are probably of particular importance in genetic mechanisms, other interactions may also be responsible for mechanisms of carcinogenesis.

Mechanisms of chemical carcinogenesis

Although there is a large amount of data on carcinogens and their interactions with cellular constituents, the underlying mechanisms of cancer initiation and promotion are not clearly understood. The somatic cell-mutation theory fits much of the data, but there are exceptions which indicate that epigenetic phenomena may be involved in some instances.

The somatic cell-mutation theory depends upon there being an interaction between the genetic material and the carcinogen, which results in a mutation (see below). Such a mutation would account for the heritable nature of tumours, their monoclonal character, the mutagenic properties of carcinogens and the evolution of malignant cells *in vivo*. However, although the majority of carcinogens are mutagens, there are some such as ethionine and thioacetamide which do not appear to be so, and it is conceivable that in some cases the original change may not be mutational. For instance, cellular interactions with a carcinogen might result in an increase in mutations by increasing error-prone repair of genetic material, rather than by being mutational in themselves.

It is also probable that a single mutation will be insufficient to initiate tumour development, which requires loss of regulation of cell growth and division. It is therefore likely that carcinogenesis is a multistep process, the first step being the interaction between the carcinogen and cellular macromolecules. This may not necessarily result in a mutation, but will result in a heritable change in phenotypic expression which involves continuous modification of the structure and function of the genetic apparatus. In support of this idea of a multistep process is the fact that some mutagenic compounds, such as sodium azide and styrene oxide, do not appear to be carcinogenic.

Epigenetic mechanisms have therefore been proposed to account for these discrepancies. For example, reversion of tumour cells from a neoplastic to a quasi-normal state may occur and has been interpreted as being indicative of an epigenetic mechanism. This would involve repression and derepression of genetic material or expression of the genotype, in an analogous fashion to differentiation being regarded as directed repression and derepression. Therefore, the interaction of carcinogens with cellular mediators of genetic expression would be a non-mutational mode of carcinogenesis. A carcinogen might also alter the response of the cell to growth controls by non-genetic effects or decrease the efficiency of the immunological surveillance system. It is also possible that both epigenetic and genetic mechanisms may be involved at various stages of tumour initiation and promotion.

The cellular targets with which carcinogens might interact are numerous, but attention has been focused on the nucleic acids, particularly DNA. It is indisputable that a number of carcinogens which are mutagenic do alkylate or arylate bases in the DNA molecules such as at the O^6 and N^7 positions of guanine (figure 6.2) and that such covalent interactions correlate well with carcinogenicity (figure 6.3). It now seems clear, however, that the specific nature of the covalent interaction is important, possibly because of the ability of the cell to repair the altered nucleic acid, and hence avoid mispairing and the incorporation of a mutation. Thus, the methylation of guanine at the O^6 position is more crucial than that at N^7, as excision repair of O^6 methyl-guanine is poor in certain tissues, these tissues being more susceptible to

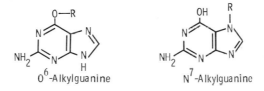

O^6-Alkylguanine N^7-Alkylguanine

Figure 6.2. O^6 and N^7 alkylation of guanine.

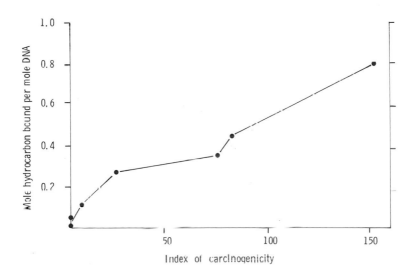

Figure 6.3. Relationship between the binding of carcinogens to DNA and carcinogenic potency. Adapted from Brookes (1966) *Cancer Res.*, **26**, 1994.

tumour development. Initiation of error-prone repair by compounds may also lead to the occurrence of mutations.

It has also been suggested that RNA and proteins might be targets for carcinogens. Recent work has indicated that residues of the carcinogen acetylaminofluorene found in ribosomal RNA may correlate more closely with liver tumour development than those residues in DNA.

Direct interactions with the mechanisms of protein synthesis or with DNA and RNA polymerase enzymes can also be seen as possible mechanisms. For instance, a modification of the polymerase enzymes by a carcinogen either directly or indirectly could lead to the erroneous replication of DNA or RNA and hence the permanent incorporation of a mutation.

In conclusion, it is clear that the mechanisms underlying chemical carcinogenesis are complex, involving numerous steps and more than a single gene mutation. It is also clear that the cell may protect itself from chemical carcinogens by repair of altered macromolecules, thereby resisting potent mutagens. Perhaps failure of these repair mechanisms leading to incorporation of mutations, coupled with epigenetic effects or the derepression of growth control, are some of the major factors involved in the initiation of cancer by chemicals.

Tissue lesions

Introduction

Some toxic substances may cause direct damage to tissues which may often be irreversible. However, the importance of the lesion depends on the particular type of tissue damaged. Thus, the degree of specialization of the cells comprising the tissue and the reserve functional capacity of the organ determine the importance of the toxic response to the whole organism. The cells of the skin and those at the sites of absorption are particularly vulnerable to the directly damaging effects of toxic compounds, as the concentration is highest at this point. Thus the cells of the skin, gastrointestinal tract and lungs may suffer local irritant damage from toxic compounds.

It is not within the scope of this book to examine the different types of tissue lesion. We shall simply look briefly at cellular damage and the organ systems most often damaged by toxic compounds.

Liver

The liver may be considered to be the portal to the tissues of the organism, the route by which orally administered compounds pass into the body, and consequently damage to the liver is a common toxic response. The liver is served by the portal vein and hepatic artery and is drained by the hepatic vein and the bile duct. The portal vein brings food and other compounds such as toxins from the gut, and the hepatic artery supplies oxygenated blood.

Classically, the hepatic architecture is divided into lobules, on the basis of the vessels mentioned above. The lobule is an area bounded by the portal tracts, consisting of the hepatic artery, portal vein and the bile duct, arranged around the central vein. The area around the portal tract is the periportal region, that around the central vein the centrilobular region and the area between these is the midzonal region (figure 6.4).

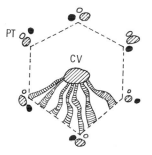

PT

CV

Figure 6.4. Schematic representation of the classic liver lobule. PT is the portal tract, which is made up of branches of the portal vein and hepatic artery and a bile duct. CV is a branch of the central vein. Adapted from Plaa, G. L. (1980) Toxic responses of the liver. In *Casarett and Doull's Toxicology, The Basic Science of Poisons*, edited by J. Doull, C. D. Klaasen and M. O. Amdur (New York: Macmillan).

More recently the liver architecture has been redescribed in terms of functional units known as acini (figure 6.5). The simple acinus is arranged around the portal space and consists of a terminal portal venule, hepatic arteriole, bile ductule, lymph vessels and nerves. There are circulatory zones within the acinus (zones 1, 2 and 3, figure 6.5) which are preferentially fed by the parent vessels of that acinus and which coincide approximately with the lobular regions (for more details see chapters by Plaa and Rappaport).

Although the majority of the liver is composed of hepatocytes, there are other cell types present, such as endothelial cells, bile duct cells, Kupfer cells, nerve cells and the cells of the connective tissue. These various cell types differ in the extent to which they are able to metabolize foreign compounds and in the protective mechanisms with which they are equipped, and they therefore vary in their susceptibility to toxic substances. The hepatocytes in the various areas of the lobule also differ in their enzymic capabilities, and consequently toxic damage may be confined to one area. For instance,

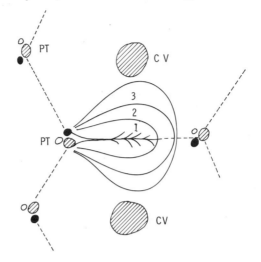

Figure 6.5. Schematic representation of a hepatic acinus. PT represents the portal tract, consisting of branches of the portal vein and hepatic artery and a bile duct. CV represents a branch of the central vein. The areas 1, 2 and 3 represent the various zones draining the terminal afferent vessel. Adapted from Rappaport, A. M. (1969). In *Diseases of the Liver*, edited by L. Schiff (Philadelphia: J. B. Lippincott).

cytochrome P-450 content is maximal in the region near to the central vein, and this is probably the major reason for the development of centrilobular necrosis after the administration of compounds which require metabolic toxication. Other enzymes, such as alcohol dehydrogenase, are located particularly in the periportal region. Compounds such as allyl alcohol (figure 4.28) specifically cause periportal necrosis due to metabolism to toxic metabolites catalysed by alcohol dehydrogenase in this area of the liver.

The liver may sustain various types and degrees of damage from toxic substances and hepatotoxins, and the lesions they produce have been variously classified by different workers in the field (see chapter by Plaa). Briefly, the types of hepatic damage are necrosis, fat accumulation, cholestasis, cirrhosis and carcinogenesis. These different lesions vary in severity and the underlying mechanisms are different. Thus, severe irreversible damage may occur which leads to cell death and necrosis, or the toxic effect may be reversible, such as the accumulation of triglycerides in fatty liver which is a common hepatic response to toxic compounds (see below). Liver damage may be an acute response following single doses or it may be due to chronic exposure, and the toxic effect after chronic exposure may be different from the acute response. For instance, ethionine (see Chapter 7) causes fatty liver after acute doses, but given chronically causes cirrhosis.

The type of liver injury produced depends on the particular toxic substance and its mode of action. Certain compounds cause periportal necrosis, whereas many produce centrilobular necrosis, in some cases because of the distribution of metabolizing enzymes as mentioned above. The degree of liver damage clearly depends on the dose, ranging from single-cell necrosis in the centrilobular region to massive necrosis throughout the liver, as is the case with carbon tetrachloride.

Toxic substances may act directly upon hepatocytes either as the parent compound or a toxic metabolite, or they may act upon a hepatic process such as bile secretion. For instance, acute doses of α-naphthylisothiocyanate reduce biliary flow and cause a cholestatic type of liver damage. It is thought that the bile salts retained as a result of the bile stasis and hyperbilirubinaemia contribute to the hepatic damage.

An alternative mechanism of hepatotoxicity may involve an immune response. For instance, one of the mechanisms proposed for the hepato-toxicity of the anaesthetic halothane involves alteration of the hepatocyte membrane by a covalent interaction with a reactive metabolite of the drug. The altered cell surface which results is antigenic and stimulates production of an antibody which renders liver cells susceptible to attack by cytotoxic lymphocytes, thereby destroying the hepatocytes.

Kidney

The blood passing through the kidney represents 20–25% of the cardiac output, and the function of the kidney is to filter out of this blood waste products and toxins. The kidney is a complex arrangement of vascular endothelial cells and tubular epithelial cells, the blood vessels and tubules being intertwined. The functional unit of the kidney is the nephron, which passes from the cortex to the medulla (figure 6.6). The environment inside and outside of the nephron varies along its length and this influences the type of toxic effect produced by nephrotoxic agents.

The kidney has a marked ability to compensate for tissue damage and loss, and consequently unless it is evaluated immediately a nephrotoxic effect may not be recognized. Similarly, chronic nephrotoxicity may not be recognized because of this compensatory ability.

Substances are concentrated, following glomerular filtration of the plasma water, in the tubular lumen by reabsorption of 98–99% of the sodium and water. The concentration of toxic substances in the tubular lumen and surrounding renal parenchymal cells may therefore be very high. The ratio of tubular fluid concentration to plasma concentration may reach values of 500 : 1. The countercurrent exchange of small molecules may lead to very high concentrations of compounds in the interstitial fluid of the renal medulla. Reabsorption of compounds from the tubular lumen may lead to high concentrations of compounds in the cells of the nephron also. For example, the antibiotics gentamycin and cephaloridine are both nephrotoxic,

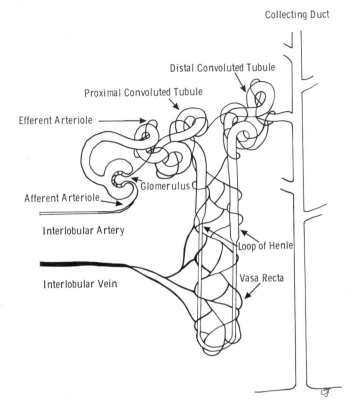

Figure 6.6. Schematic representation of a mammalian nephron.

seemingly by being accumulated in the cells of the proximal tubule. Cephaloridine nephrotoxicity may also involve metabolic activation of the drug, but whether this is renal or hepatic metabolism is unclear.

It is therefore clear that the tissues of the kidney are often exposed to higher concentrations of potentially toxic compounds than most other tissues. In many cases the metabolites are less toxic and more polar and water-soluble than the parent compound, and the higher concentrations in the kidney do not result in toxicity. If the metabolite excreted is more toxic, however, the kidney is in a particularly vulnerable position.

The pH of the lumen tends towards acidity, and this may cause hydrolysis of metabolites or changes in their solubility. For example, some of the early sulphonamides, which were given in high doses, were found to cause renal tubular necrosis. In some cases this was due to crystallization of the less soluble acetylated metabolites (table 4.1) in the lumen of the tubule with consequent irritation of the surrounding cells and eventual necrosis.

It is clear that there are many mechanisms underlying nephrotoxicity. These range from the simple irritant or abrasive effects of high concentrations of foreign compounds such as sulphonamides giving rise to tubular necrosis, to the ischaemic injury of the tubular structures proposed to underly aspirin-induced medullary lesions. The latter has been suggested as being due to inhibition of prostaglandin synthesis by aspirin, giving rise to vasospasm in the vasa recta and hence reduction of blood flow resulting in ischaemia (figure 6.7).

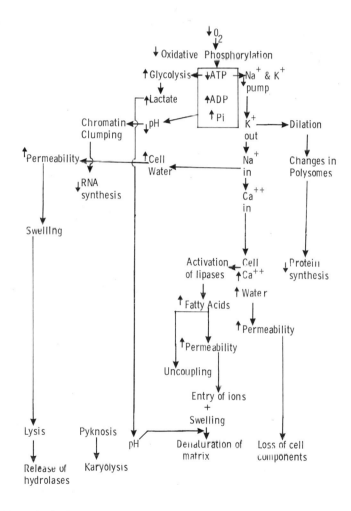

Figure 6.7. Hypothetical sequence of events leading to a necrotic cell following ischaemic cell injury. Small vertical arrows denote an increase (↑) or decrease (↓). Adapted from Trump, B. F. & Arstila, A. U. (1975). In *Principles of Pathobiology*, edited by M. F. La Via and R. B. Hill (New York: Oxford University Press).

Lung

The lung is an organ in a particularly vulnerable position as regards toxic substances, as it may be involved in both the absorption and excretion of volatile toxins. Furthermore, it may also suffer selective damage from non-volatile toxic compounds administered by other routes, by virtue of localization, as in the case of paraquat and ipomeanol pulmonary toxicity (see page 200).

The air of our environment is contaminated with many different potentially toxic substances: irritant gases such as sulphur dioxide, particles of dust, of metals and of other substances such as asbestos, solvents and other chemicals which may be local irritants. The lungs have a large surface area and compounds may consequently be absorbed very rapidly if they are small enough to pass through pores in the alveolar membrane (8–10 Å radius) or are lipid-soluble and able to cross the membrane by diffusion. Solid particles may be taken up by pinocytosis in some cases.

Fortunately, however, the lungs are equipped with defence mechanisms. Most of the respiratory system is lined with ciliated cells and mucus is secreted and lines the airways. Therefore, solid particles are removed by the movement of the cilia and mucus, and volatile compounds and substances in solution and inhaled as aerosols may dissolve in the mucus and be transported out of the lungs by the action of the cilia.

As an organ the lung is capable of metabolizing many foreign compounds, carrying out both phase 1 and phase 2 reactions. However, the capacity relative to the liver varies with the species, enzyme, substrate and cell type. For instance, biphenyl hydroxylase activity is slightly higher in rabbit lung compared to liver tissue, whereas the activity in rat lung is much lower than that in liver. Aniline hydroxylase and glucuronyl transferase activities are lower in rabbit lung relative to the hepatic enzyme. The non-ciliated bronchiolar cell or Clara cell is known to have mixed-function oxidase activity, metabolizing ipomeanol to a reactive metabolite which causes lung damage. Thus, although the lung is able to detoxify foreign compounds this example shows that toxication may also occur.

There are over 40 different cell types in the respiratory system (see chapter by Menzel and McClellan). Those cells particularly susceptible to injury are the lining cells of trachea and bronchi, endothelial cells and the interstitial cells (fibroblasts and fibrocytes).

Some toxic substances, such as sulphur dioxide, nitrogen dioxide and ozone, may cause acute, direct damage to lung tissue, whereas others, such as nickel carbonyl, may cause tumour formation. The types of toxic response shown by the lungs are briefly discussed below.

Irritation

The initial response to volatile irritants such as ammonia and chlorine is bronchoconstriction. These two gases are water-soluble and are absorbed in the aqueous secretions in the upper airways of the respiratory system, and do not cause residual chronic pulmonary damage. Other irritants such as arsenic compounds may cause bronchitis.

Lining-cell damage

Damage to the cells lining the airways and alveoli may lead to an increase in permeability and necrosis. This results in a release of fluid, leading to oedema. The site of this type of damage depends on the compound. If the toxic substance is volatile and has low water solubility, such as nitrogen dioxide and ozone, the effect occurs in the alveoli and small respiratory bronchioles. More water-soluble compounds may be toxic to cells higher up the airways in the trachea or bronchi.

Nitrogen dioxide and ozone cause peroxidation of cellular membranes and phosgene destroys the permeability of the alveolar cell membrane following hydrolysis to carbon dioxide and hydrogen chloride in the aqueous environment of the alveolus. (Also, as phosgene itself is a very reactive chemical, it could react directly with cellular constituents.) The increased permeability leads to fluid release and oedema. The solvent tetrachloroethylene causes necrosis and oedema in lung tissue following metabolic activation by the microsomal enzymes.

Fibrosis

This response, caused by substances such as silica (silicosis) and asbestos (asbestosis) is thought to involve the uptake of particles by macrophages. This is followed by rupture of the lysosomes, release of the enzymes contained therein and digestion of the macrophage by these enzymes. This cycle then releases the original particle and the process starts again. The result is aggregation of lymphoid tissue and stimulation of collagen formation, leading to the fibrotic lesions.

Stimulation of an allergic response

Micro-organisms, spores, dusts such as cotton dust, and certain chemicals may produce an allergic-type response with pulmonary symptoms. For instance, toluene di-isocyanate, a chemical used in the plastics industry, causes an allergic type of reaction when inhaled. It is thought to form conjugates with proteins which act as antigens (see page 159).

Pulmonary cancer

Many different materials produce tumours on inhalation. Asbestos, poly-cyclic aromatic hydrocarbons, cigarette smoke and nickel carbonyl are a few examples. Whether carcinogens such as the polycyclic aromatic hydro-carbons are metabolically activated in lung tissue or whether they are metabolized elsewhere and transported to the lungs is not clear at present. Although microsomal enzymes are present in lung tissue, the level of activity relative to liver tissue varies and, depending on the substrate, may be similar to that in the liver or perhaps one tenth of it. It is clear that the activity of the microsomal enzymes in the lung varies with the type of cell, with some, such as the Clara cell, having more activity than other cell types (see page 201).

Some compounds are pulmonary toxins when given by other routes, for example hydrazine given intraperitoneally causes lung tumours, paraquat taken orally causes lung fibrosis, probably by being actively taken up by the Type II pneumocyte cells, and ipomeanol given intraperitoneally causes necrosis of the Clara cells, as discussed in Chapter 7.

Mechanism and response in cellular injury

The direct toxic action of substances on cells may lead to irreversible damage followed by cell death. This is followed by degenerative changes such as autolysis, which involve hydrolysis of cell components and denaturation of proteins. These events constitute necrosis. Whether a cell survives a toxic insult or dies and undergoes necrosis depends on the severity of disruption and whether the cell passes the point of no return. Cellular necrosis is characterized by changes in the appearance of the cell, such as the swelling of the mitochondria, the appearance of vacuoles and the accumulation of fluid in intracellular compartments, known as hydropic degeneration. Positively charged cytoplasmic proteins increase, with a consequent increase in eosin binding or eosiniphilia, but a decrease in haematoxylin binding or basophilia. There appear to be three important features involved in cellular injury, altered cell volume regulation, altered energy metabolism, and the appearance of lysosomes or the suicide bag concept.

Altered cell volume regulation. The permeability of the plasma membrane around the cell allows ions to pass into and out of the cell. The high concen-tration of negatively charged protein relative to the extracellular environ-ment means that positively charged ions and solutes pass into the cell, with consequent expansion, unless the ions are actively transported out. This active transport is, of course, energy-dependent, requiring ATP and involving an ATPase enzyme in the membrane. The balance achieved between active transport and diffusion, allowing K^+ and Mg^{2+} into the cell but removing Na^+ and Ca^{2+}, maintains the cellular volume in equilibrium. However, the system depends on the integrity of the membrane and its enzyme systems as well as on a supply of energy. Damage to either or both may lead to a change in Na^+ and K^+ transport and isosmotic swelling, with subsequent cellular damage.

Altered energy metabolism. The production of energy within the mitochondria is closely linked with the structure. Therefore, changes in function may be accompanied by structural changes such as swelling or contraction which may be the result of the uptake of water and be the basis of hydropic degeneration. Mitochondria normally undergo low-amplitude swelling and contraction with changes in oxidative phosphorylation, and this may reflect, to some extent, the movement of water between inner and outer compartments. When water moves into the inner compartment from the outer, in high-amplitude swelling, the inner compartment expands and the cristae in the mitochondrion unfold. The membranes may rupture and then the outer compartment expands. This may be due to increased permeability.

Increases in the ratio of ADP to ATP are reflected in the contraction of the mitochondrion, such as after anoxia or the administration of electron transport inhibitors. Prolonged contraction leads to deterioration of the inner membrane and high-amplitude swelling results. Eventually, contraction becomes impossible with the rupture and deterioration of the membranes.

The appearance of lysosomes. The lysosomes contain a number of hydrolytic enzymes which, if released, may damage cell constituents. However, it seems that bursting out of the lysosomes is generally a terminal phase of injury, occurring after the point of no return has been reached, rather than a cause.

As well as direct toxic action, indirect effects such as vascular changes leading to anoxia and congestion may also be initiating events. Thus, acute ischaemia or reduction in blood supply causes necrosis of the affected tissue, and its pathogenesis is illustrative of the cellular response to injury (figure 6.7). The major changes involve changes in cellular volume and mitochondrial function.

Direct damage to the cell membrane may result from a toxic insult with consequent changes in its permeability and transport mechanisms. The changes in intracellular ion concentration which follow may result in calcification of the mitochondria due to the influx of Ca^{2+} coupled with phosphate accumulation. For instance, mercuric chloride is a nephrotoxic compound (see Chapter 7). The mercury binds to membrane sulphydryl groups and this causes a change in membrane permeability. Inactivation of the membrane transport system results and shifts in the concentration of ions occur. These ionic changes result in calcification of the mitochondria in the tubular epithelial cells (figure 6.6) and the cells become necrotic. Methyl mercury acts similarly on cell membranes in the central nervous system, and *p*-mercuribenzoate reacts with membrane sulphydryl groups and causes tissue necrosis and mitochondrial calcification.

Accumulation of triglycerides

A common reaction to cellular injury, particularly in the liver, is the accumulation of lipid in the cytoplasm. When this occurs in hepatocytes it is termed fatty liver, which is a reversible toxic response, much less severe than necrosis.

Lipids and fatty acids are taken up by the liver from the plasma and lipids may then be converted to lipoproteins for transport out of the cell. Any imbalance between the supply, utilization and secretion of lipid leads to fatty liver (figure 6.8). Thus, inhibition of protein synthesis, disturbances of phospholipid metabolism or fatty acid oxidation in mitochondria may all lead to fatty liver.

As will be discussed in Chapter 7, carbon tetrachloride and ethionine both cause fatty liver by inhibiting protein synthesis and therefore secretion of triglycerides out of the liver. Hydrazine (figure 2.1) also causes fatty liver, but

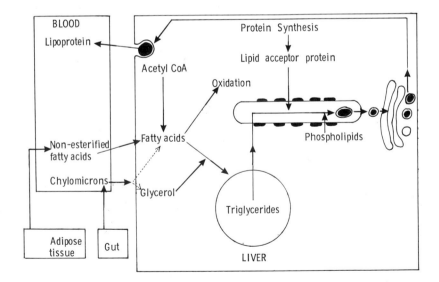

Figure 6.8. Pathways involved in lipid metabolism and distribution. Adapted from Trump, B. F. & Arstila, A. U. (1980). In *Principles of Pathobiology*, edited by M. F. La Via and R. B. Hill (New York: Oxford University Press).

by a different mechanism, probably involving increased uptake and increased intracellular synthesis of lipids.

Lipid peroxidation

One of the basic mechanisms thought to underly toxic tissue damage in some cases is lipid peroxidation. It has been implicated in the toxicities of a number of compounds, such as the hepatic necrosis caused by carbon tetrachloride and white phosphorus, the pulmonary damage due to para-quat, the destruction of the pancreatic β-cells by alloxan and the destruction of nerve terminals by 6-hydroxydopamine.

The process of lipid peroxidation may be initiated by direct attack of a foreign free radical on unsaturated lipids or the reaction of singlet oxygen or hydroxyl radicals generated by foreign compounds. The result is a chain reaction which, in the presence of oxygen, is terminated with the production of lipid alcohols, lipid aldehydes and the oxidative destruction of cellular lipids. (A free radical is a molecular species which has an unpaired electron. It is formed by homolytic cleavage of a covalent bond, either spontaneously or following irradiation, by addition of an electron or by the abstraction of a hydrogen atom by another radical.)

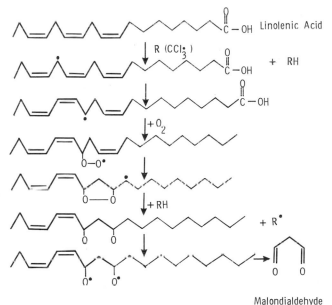

Malondialdehyde

Figure 6.9. Peroxidative destruction of a polyunsaturated lipid initiated by a free radical attack such as by the trichloromethyl radical ($CCl_3^{\bullet}$). Adapted from Slater, T. F. (1972) *Free Radicals in Tissue Injury* (London: Pion).

Polyunsaturated fatty acids, found particularly in the membranes of subcellular organelles, are especially susceptible to free radical attack, such as from the trichloromethyl radical derived metabolically from carbon tetrachloride. The types of reaction which may occur are shown in figure 6.9. These chain reactions may be propagated throughout the cell. The final products of the oxidative breakdown of lipids are various lipid alcohols and aldehydes and very short-chain products such as malondialdehyde (figure 6.9). Some of these are toxic to the cell and distribute the toxic effects away from the initial point of attack, which may be the endoplasmic reticulum as it is in carbon tetrachloride hepatotoxicity.

The effects of lipid peroxidation are numerous and complex. The structural integrity of lipids in membranes is adversely affected, leading to damage to some structures. Cross-linking may occur between lipids and between lipids and proteins, which may alter the structure and function of membranes and intracellular organelles. For example, lipid peroxidation may damage the lysosomal membrane, leading to disruption of this organelle and the loss of the contents. The hydrolytic enzymes released cause intracellular damage. Sulphydryl groups are particularly susceptible to lipid peroxidation, and enzymes which contain them may show loss of activity if the products of lipid peroxidation react with them.

However, not all compounds causing tissue damage initiate lipid peroxidation. For example, thioacetamide- and chloroform-induced liver damage do not seem to involve lipid peroxidation, and therefore it is not a general mechanism underlying all cellular damage.

Protective mechanisms

Biological systems possess a number of mechanisms whereby they may protect themselves against toxic foreign compounds, and some of these have already been mentioned. For instance, metabolic transformation to more polar metabolites which are readily excreted is one method of detoxication, and hence protection, already discussed. Thus, conjugation of a phenol such as paracetamol with glucuronic acid or sulphate facilitates excretion of the drug and diverts the compound away from potentially toxic pathways (see Chapter 7).

Probably the most important detoxication or protective mechanism of this type is conjugation with the tripeptide glutathione as discussed in Chapter 4. Glutathione conjugation is of major importance in detoxifying reactive compounds. Sufficiently reactive substances may react directly with glutathione, whereas other reactions may only take place when catalysed by one of the glutathione transferase enzymes. A wide variety of compounds react with glutathione either with or without the help of enzymes and are thereby detoxified and excreted in the bile, or in the urine as mercapturic acids after further metabolism. Compounds which react with glutathione may be chemically reactive intermediates formed metabolically, such as aromatic, aliphatic or heterocyclic epoxides, which are in some cases capable of tissue damage at the site of metabolism. Alternatively, other compounds which react with glutathione are chemically stable and relatively non-toxic, such as diethyl maleate, used experimentally to deplete hepatic glutathione *in vivo*.

Another important protective mechanism of this type is the hydration of epoxides catalysed by epoxide hydratase (see page 71). This metabolic route is of particular importance, for instance, in the toxicity of bromobenzene, where the action of epoxide hydratase diverts the toxic, reactive epoxide away from reaction with tissue proteins (see page 194).

Apart from protective mechanisms which involve detoxication by metabolism as described, there are mechanisms which protect the cell against secondary products of exposure to toxic substances. For instance, superoxide anion radical (O_2^-; the result of a one-electron reduction of molecular oxygen) is thought to be produced by the herbicide paraquat and to be involved in the pathogenesis of the lung lesions produced by this toxin. Other secondary toxic products are hydrogen peroxide, hydroxyl radicals, lipid radicals and lipid hydroperoxides. The production of some of these has been mentioned in the section on lipid peroxidation and in the discussion of carbon tetrachloride hepatotoxicity. These secondary products may be detoxified in a number of ways.

Superoxide anion radical is removed by the enzyme superoxide dismutase which catalyses the reaction·

$$O_2^- + O_2^- + 2H \longrightarrow O_2 + H_2O_2$$

Lipid radicals and other radicals may be removed by a number of endogenous compounds, including glutathione. Others are ascorbate, vitamin K, vitamin E (α-tocopherol) and cysteine. These compounds act as alternative hydrogen donors to the allylic hydrogen atoms of unsaturated lipids. α-Tocopherol is thought to be involved in the protection of organisms against a number of toxic substances, and consequently vitamin E deficiency enhances the toxicity of such substances, paraquat for example.

α-Tocopherol (TH) reacts with lipid hydroperoxide radicals:

$$L\cdot + O_2 \longrightarrow LO_2\cdot$$

Propagation $\quad LO_2\cdot + LH \longrightarrow LOOH + L\cdot$

Antioxidant $\quad LO_2\cdot + \alpha TH \longrightarrow LOOH + \alpha T\cdot$

Termination $\quad LO_2\cdot + \alpha T\cdot \longrightarrow LOOH + \alpha TQ$

The final products are lipid hydroperoxides and α-tocopherol quinone (TQ).

Another important protective mechanism is the glutathione peroxidase system. Reduced glutathione reacts with radicals, reduces unstable and reactive lipid hydroperoxides to lipid alcohols and reduces hydrogen peroxide to water. The oxidized glutathione produced by these reactions is reduced by NADPH, generated from glucose-6-phosphate dehydrogenase and glucose-6-phosphate (see chapters by Bus, Gibson and Slater).

Physiological or pharmacodynamic effects

Toxic foreign compounds may affect the homeostasis of an organism by altering basic biochemical processes, and such effects may often be reversible if inhibition of an enzyme or binding to a receptor is involved. A well defined dose–response is often observed with such effects, and the end-point may be the death of the animal if a process of central importance is affected.

The inhibition of enzymes, blockade of receptors or changes in membrane permeability which underly these physiological responses often rely on reversible interactions. These are dependent upon the concentration of the toxic compound at the site of action and possibly the concentration of an endogenous substrate, if competitive inhibition is involved. Therefore, with the loss of the toxic compound from the body, by the processes of metabolism and excretion, the concentration at the site of action falls and the normal function of the receptor or enzyme returns. This is in direct contrast to the type of toxic effect in which a cellular structure or macromolecule is permanently damaged or altered by the foreign compound. It should be noted, however, that in some cases a severe physiological disturbance, such as prolonged anoxia, may allow irreversible changes to take place within the cell.

There are many different types of physiological response, with a variety of mechanisms, and it is not within the scope of this book to examine these mechanisms in detail. However, an illustration of some of the various types of physiological change that may be encountered as toxic responses is instructive as these are probably the most frequently encountered type of adverse drug effects in clinical practice. In many cases the basic biochemical mechanisms underlying such effects are not understood and involve the complex interrelationships of various control processes. The following are examples of the types of physiological response that may be caused by a foreign compound. They may involve effects on major organs or on general physiological mechanisms.

Anoxia

Lack of oxygen in the tissues may be due to respiratory or circulatory failure, or be caused directly by compounds such as carbon monoxide binding to haemoglobin, instead of oxygen.

Inhibition of cellular respiration

This type of effect occurs in all tissues, being caused by metabolic inhibitors such as cyanide, which inhibits the electron transport chain. Inhibition of one or more of the enzymes of the tricarboxylic acid cycle, such as that by fluoroacetate (see Chapter 7) also results in inhibition of cellular respiration (figure 7.23).

Respiratory failure

Excessive muscular blockade may be caused by compounds such as the cholinesterase inhibitors. Such inhibitors, exemplified by the organophosphate insecticides (e.g. malathion, figure 7.18) and nerve gases (e.g. isopropylmethylphosphonofluoridate) cause death by blockade of respiratory muscles secondary to excess acetylcholine accumulation. This is due to inhibition of the enzymes normally responsible for the inactivation of this neurotransmitter (see page 206).

Disturbances of the central nervous system

Drugs and toxic substances which interfere with normal neurotransmission may cause central effects. For example, cholinesterase inhibitors such as the organophosphate insecticides (e.g. malathion, figure 7.18) cause the accumulation of excess acetylcholine. The accumulation of this neurotransmitter in the central nervous system in humans exposed to such toxic insecticides leads to anxiety, restlessness, insomnia, slurred speech, convulsions and depression of the respiratory and circulatory centres.

Hyper/hypotension

Drastic changes in blood pressure may occur as a toxic response to a foreign compound, such as the hypotension caused by hydrazoic acid and sodium azide. There may be various mechanisms, such as vasodilation, β-adrenoceptor blockade or altered water balance.

Hyper/hypoglycaemia

Changes in blood sugar concentration may be caused by foreign compounds. Drugs such as tolbutamide, a sulphonylurea, are used therapeutically to lower blood sugar levels. Streptozotocin, which is used to treat pancreatic cancer, damages the β-cells in the pancreas and this leads to hyperglycaemia. The industrial chemical hydrazine (figure 5.19), which is highly toxic, causes hypoglycaemia.

Anaesthesia

The induction of unconsciousness may be the result of exposure to excessive amounts of toxic solvents such as carbon tetrachloride, as well as to clinically used volatile and non-volatile anaesthetics such as halothane and thiopental. The mechanism(s) underlying anaesthesia are not fully understood, although there have been numerous theories. Many of these have centred on the correlation between certain physical properties and anaesthetic potency. Thus, the oil: water partition coefficient, ability to reduce surface tension and to induce the formation of clathrate compounds with water are all correlated with anaesthetic potency. These are all related to the physical factors which determine hydrophobicity. The site of action may therefore be a hydrophobic region in a membrane or protein.

Changes in water and electrolyte balance

Certain foreign compounds may cause the retention or excretion of water. Some, such as the drug furosemide, are used therapeutically as diuretics. Other compounds causing diuresis are ethanol, caffeine and certain mercury compounds, such as mersalyl. Diuresis may be the result of a direct effect on the kidney, as with mercury compounds which inhibit the reabsorption of chloride, whereas other diuretics such as ethanol influence the production of antidiuretic hormone by the pituitary.

Ion transport

Alteration of the movement of ions such as potassium in heart tissue may be a toxic response to some foreign compounds. For example, the digitalis glycosides cause changes in tissue potassium and this may lead to serious cardiac effects.

Failure of energy supply

Toxic compounds which interfere with major pathways in intermediary metabolism may lead to depletion of energy-rich intermediates. For example, fluoroacetate blocks the tricarboxylic acid cycle, giving rise to cardiac and central nervous system effects which may be fatal (see Chapter 7, figure 7.23).

Changes in muscle—contraction/relaxation

This type of response may be caused by several mechanisms. For instance, the muscle relaxation induced by succinylcholine, discussed in more detail later, is due to blockade of neuromuscular transmission. Alternatively, acetylcholine antagonists such as tubocurarine may compete for the receptor site at the skeletal muscle end plate, leading to paralysis of the skeletal muscle.

Hypo/hyperthermia

Certain foreign compounds can cause changes in body temperature which may become a toxic reaction if they are extreme. Antipyretic drugs such as aspirin lower body temperature, other foreign compounds may cause hyperthermia. An example of the latter is 2,4-dinitrophenol, which uncouples oxidative phosphorylation in the mitochondria, thereby allowing energy to be released as heat instead of producing ATP for metabolic processes.

Heightened sensitivity

Heightened sensitivity may be caused by a foreign compound. For instance, exposure to certain halogenated hydrocarbons, such as the fluorocarbons used in aerosol sprays, may sensitize heart muscle to endogenous catecholamines. This sensitization, in some cases following intentional inhalation, has resulted in sudden death from heart failure.

Teratogenesis

Introduction

Teratogenesis involves interference with the normal development of either the embryo or foetus *in utero*, giving rise to abnormalities in the neonate. This interference may take many forms and there is therefore no general mechanism underlying this type of response. Many of the toxic effects described elsewhere in this book may be teratogenic in the appropriate circumstances.

Teratogenic agents may be drugs taken during pregnancy, radiation, both ionizing and non-ionizing, environmental pollutants, chemical hazards in the workplace, dietary deficiencies and natural contaminants.

Although mutations occurring in germ cells may give rise to abnormalities in the neonate, such as Down's syndrome, teratogenicity is normally confined to the effect of foreign agents on somatic cells within either the developing embryo or foetus and the consequent effects on that individual, rather than inherited defects. However, the effects of foreign compounds on germ cells will also be considered within the context of teratogenesis in this section.

Embryogenesis is a very complex process involving cell proliferation, differentiation, migration and organogenesis. This sequence of events (figure 6.10) is controlled by information transcribed and translated from DNA and RNA respectively (figure 6.15) in a time-dependent manner.

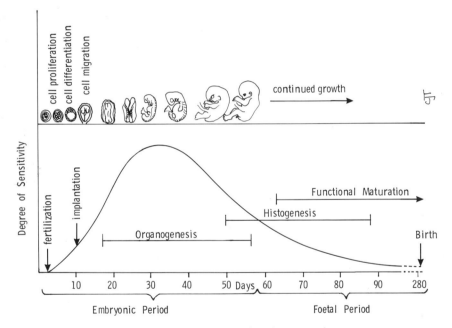

Figure 6.10. The stages of embryogenesis.

Although embryogenesis is not fully understood and is a highly complex process, with the knowledge available certain predictions may be made regarding teratogenesis:

(*a*) The sequence of events in embryogenesis could be easily disturbed, its interrelationships readily disrupted and such interference could be very specific;

(*b*) The timing of the interference with the process of embryogenesis would be very important to the final expression of the teratogenic effect.

Both of these predictions are found to be correct, and the teratogenic effect may be out of all proportion to the initiating event, if this event occurs at a critical time. This teratogenic effect might simply be a slowing down in the development of one group of cells, which are then out of synchrony with the overall process of embryonic development. For example, a deficiency of folic acid in pregnant rats may cause reno-uteral defects in the neonate because migration of certain primordial cell groups is disturbed by this deficiency. The cell groups are then not able to attain their correct position at a later stage.

A further prediction might be that any effect or foreign compound which interfered with biochemical pathways, particularly transcription and translation, damaged macromolecules, caused a deficiency of essential cofactors, caused a reduction in energy supply or produced direct tissue damage, would probably be teratogenic. Thus ionizing radiation, which causes mutations and other effects, will readily cause birth defects if the pregnant animal is irradiated at the appropriate time. Pre-existing mutations derived from the maternal or paternal germ cells may also result in mutations, of course.

The mechanisms underlying teratogenesis are therefore many and varied, and true understanding will only come with greater understanding of the remarkable but complex process of embryogenesis. However, the characteristics of teratogenesis can be examined and general mechanisms described.

Characteristics of teratogenesis

Selectivity

Teratogens interfere with either embryonic or foetal development, but often do not affect the placenta or maternal organism. They are therefore selectively either embryotoxic or foetotoxic, giving rise to manifestations of such toxicity up to and including death, with subsequent abortion. The most potent teratogens may be regarded as those with no observable toxicity to the maternal system, but causing malformations in the foetus rather than death, such as the now infamous drug thalidomide. Clearly, most teratogens will cause foetal death at high enough doses and probably maternal toxicity also. Certain compounds, such as colchicine, which cause foetal death do not cause malformations, however.

Genetic influences

Observations that species and strain differences exist in the susceptibility to certain teratogens suggests that genetic factors may be involved in teratogenesis. Similarly, it seems clear that in some cases at least a teratogen may increase the frequency of a naturally occurring abnormality. These genetic factors may simply be differences in the maternal metabolism or distribution of the compound which lead to variation in the exposure to the ultimate teratogenic agent.

It is also clear from the previous discussion, however, that the instructions for the complex series of events which constitute organogenesis are probably coded in DNA, and consequently mutations or damage to DNA will be expected to cause certain abnormalities if that information is transcribed and translated. Also, genetic susceptibility to mutation or chromosome breakage may be factors. For example, the vitamin antagonist 6-amino-nicotinamide causes cleft palate and chromosomal abnormalities in mice. The chromosomal abnormalities are found in the somatic cells of a number of tissues, leading to faulty mitosis. This is supported by the fact that in some cases only one or two embryos are malformed out of several in multiparous animals, and this indicates that the embryonic genotype may sometimes be an important factor. However, although many mutagens and carcinogens are teratogenic, not all are, suggesting that genetic factors are not always involved in the underlying mechanisms of teratogenesis.

Susceptibility and development stage

The susceptibility of both an embryo and a foetus to a teratogen is variable, depending on the stage of development when exposure occurs. For gross anatomical abnormalities the critical periods of organogenesis are the most susceptible to exposure, whereas other types of abnormality may have other critical periods for exposure.

After fertilization, the cells divide, giving rise to a blastocyst. During this time there is little morphological differentiation of cells, except that some are located on the surfaces and others internally. The development of the blastocyst gives an internal cavity (the blastocoele) and hence further surfaces and positional differences. However, there are few specific teratogenic effects which occur at this time, the major effects being death or overall developmental retardation.

The appearance of the embryonic germ layers, the ectoderm, endoderm and mesoderm is the next stage, with the gross segregation of cells into groups. Damage at this stage may be associated with specific effects.

The chemical determination which precedes structural differentiation is still not understood but it is probable that this period is sensitive to interference.

Organogenesis, which is the segregation of cells, cell groups and tissues into primordia destined to be organs is particularly sensitive to teratogens although not exclusively so. Histological differentiation occurs concurrently with, and continues after, organogenesis, as does acquisition of function. Both of these stages may be susceptible to teratogens, and exposure to them may lead to defects, although generally these defects are not gross structural ones.

The sensitive period for induction of malformations is the 5-14 day period in the rat and mouse and the 3rd week to the 3rd month in humans. This is illustrated in figure 6.11 for the teratogen actinomycin D. The later period of foetal development, like the initial proliferative stage, is less susceptible to specific effects and an 'all or none' type of response is usually seen, such as either death or no gross effect.

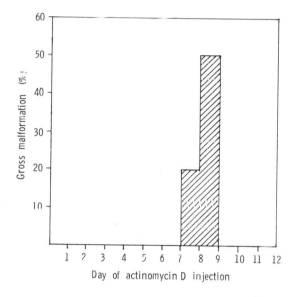

Figure 6.11. Critical timing of the teratogenic effects of actinomycin D in the rat. The histogram shows the percentage of gross malformations among surviving foetuses after a dose of 75 µg/kg, i.p. Adapted from Tuchmann-Duplessis & Mercier-Parot (1960). *Congenital Malformations*, Ciba Foundation Symposium, edited by G. E. W. Wolstenholme and C. M. O'Connor (Boston: Little Brown).

Specificity

Different types of teratogens may give similar abnormalities if given during the same critical periods. Therefore, the particular abnormality may represent interference with a specific developmental process (figure 6.12). Although there is a wide variety of possible biochemical effects or structural changes at the molecular level, these may be manifested as relatively few types of abnormal embryogenesis and hence similar defects may result from different teratogens. Thus, excessive cell death, incorrect cellular interaction,

F

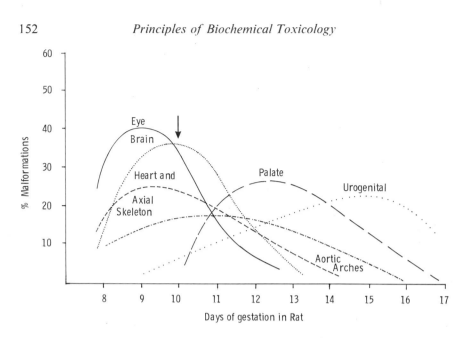

Figure 6.12. Periods of peak sensitivity to teratogens in the rat. A teratogen administered at the time shown by the arrow would cause a mixture of malformations. It would particularly damage the eyes and brain but would have little or no effect on the palate. Adapted from Wilson, J. G. (1973) *Environment and Birth Defects* (New York: Academic Press).

reduced biosynthesis of RNA, DNA or protein might be the primary manifestations of the teratogenic effect, but all give rise to the impaired migration of cells or cell groups. The eventual effect might conceivably be too few cells or cell products at a particular site for normal morphogenesis or maturation to proceed.

Manifestations of abnormal development

The final consequences of abnormal development are death, malformation, growth retardation and functional disorder. Each of these consequences follows exposure at different stages. Thus foetal death may result from exposure at an early or late stage of development to high concentrations of the toxin, without evidence of malformation. This may be due to substantial damage to the undifferentiated cells in the early stages or interference with some physiological mechanism in the late stage of development.

Malformations tend to occur following exposure during organogenesis, whereas functional disorders would be expected at later stages. The period of foetal growth is susceptible and agents acting at this time may cause growth retardation. Growth retardation may reflect a variety of functional deficiencies and both of these may occur without any sign of malformations.

Access to the embryo and foetus

For foreign compounds, in contrast to ionizing and other radiation or mechanical force, the route of access is via the maternal body. This is either through the fluids surrounding the embryo or via the blood, following the formation of the placenta. Therefore, the concentration of the compound in the embryo or foetus is dependent on the concentration in the maternal blood. The exposure of the embryo and foetus is governed by the maternal ability to excrete and metabolize the foreign compound, reflected in the plasma concentration and half-life. Most unbound compounds readily cross the placenta, if they are of low molecular weight (less than 600) and not highly charged. This passage may occur by diffusion (simple or facilitated), active transport or pinocytosis.

Metabolism of the compound may occur in the foetus, and this may lead to a prolonged foetal half-life if the metabolite is a more polar compound.

Dose–response

There clearly seems to be a 'no effect' level for most if not all teratogens with regard to death and malformations. This is probably also the case for growth retardation, but there is little evidence on which to base a firm conclusion regarding functional deficiences. It is clear that a critical number of cells have to be damaged before an effect is manifested. It can be demonstrated that there is a dose–response relation between the number of cells affected and the final degree of embryotoxicity. Most foreign compounds can be shown to be embryotoxic if given in sufficient doses at the appropriate time.

For some teratogens, the dose–response for embryotoxicity is very different from that for lethality, whereas for others there is a close parallelism. For instance, thalidomide is only embryolethal at several times the dose required to produce malformations, whereas actinomycin D is embryolethal at the lowest teratogenic dose (see page 217, figure 7.28).

Mechanisms of teratogenesis

The initiating events underlying the abnormal development or death of the foetus usually occur at the subcellular or molecular level and consequently are not readily detectable until demonstrable as cell death or tissue disruption.

The types of underlying mechanisms involved can be briefly described, however.

Mutation

It is clear that mutations are the basis of many errors of development; maybe 20–30% of those occurring in humans are due to heritable mutations in the germ line. Mutations may occur in the genetic material of either the germ cells or the somatic cells. Germ cell mutations are heritable, whereas effects in somatic cells are only apparent in the foetus exposed. Somatic cell mutations will probably not lead to gross manifestations of damage such as malformations, unless a sufficiently large number of progeny cells are affected. Consequently, somatic cell mutations are probably an infrequent cause of foetal abnormality. Some somatic mutations, however, may be incompatible with the viability of the affected cell or group of cells. This might be less damaging than a viable mutant cell which was the ancestor of an important organ or structure, however. Although some mutagens such as alkylating agents are also teratogens, there seems to be only limited overlap between them.

Chromosomal aberrations

Aberrations in chromosomes or chromatids which are sometimes microscopically visible may arise during mitotic division when newly divided chromosomes fail to separate or do so incorrectly. The absence of a chromosome is usually lethal, and an excess is often poorly tolerated, giving rise to serious defects. Aberrations of the sex chromosomes are more readily tolerated, however. Chromosome aberrations may be caused by foreign compounds as indicated in the section on mutagenesis (see page 169).

Mitotic interference

Interference with spindle formation, inhibition or arrest of DNA synthesis or the incorrect separation of chromatids all fall into this category. Inhibition of DNA synthesis, such as that caused by cytosine arabinoside, slows or arrests mitosis, which cannot progress beyond the S-phase. Inhibition of spindle formation such as that caused by vincristine or colchicine stops separation of chromosomes at anaphase (see page 170). Proper separation of chromatids may not occur because of 'stickiness' or bridging between the chromatids.

Interference with nucleic acids

A number of antineoplastic and antibiotic drugs which interfere with nucleic acid function are teratogenic. Such effects as changes in replication, transcription, the incorporation of bases and translation occurring in somatic cells are non-heritable and may be embryotoxic. Interference with protein synthesis is generally lethal to the embryo rather than malformation-causing.

Examples of teratogenic compounds which interfere with nucleic acid metabolism are cytosine arabinoside, which inhibits DNA polymerase, mitomycin C, which causes cross-linking, and 6-mercaptopurine, which blocks the incorporation of the precursors, adenylate and guanylate. Actinomycin D, a well known teratogen, intercalates with DNA and binds deoxyguanosine, interfering with RNA transcription and causing erroneous base incorporation. 8-Azaguanine is a teratogenic analogue of guanine.

Compounds such as puromycin and cycloheximide, which block rRNA transfer, and streptomycin and lincomycin, which cause misreading of mRNA, block protein synthesis and are therefore often embryolethal.

Substrate deficiency

If the requirements for the growth and development of the foetus are withheld, a disruption to these processes may occur and damage may ensue. Deficiencies in essential substrates, such as folic acid, may be caused by dietary lack or by substrate analogues.

Failure in the placental transport of essential substrates may be teratogenic and can be caused by certain compounds such as azo dyes. This has, however, only been demonstrated in rodents because of the inverted yolk sac type of placenta such animals have.

Deficiency of vitamins, such as folic acid, is highly teratogenic, as essential synthetic metabolic pathways are blocked or reduced. This may be caused by the administration of specific vitamin analogues or antagonists as well as by a failure in supply.

Deficiency of energy supply

The rapidly proliferating and differentiating tissue of the embryo would be expected to require high levels of energy, and therefore interference with its supply, not suprisingly, may be a teratogenic action. A deficiency of glucose due to dietary factors or due to hypoglycaemia, which may be induced by foreign compounds, is teratogenic. Interference in glycolysis, such as that caused by 6-aminonicotinamide, inhibition of the tricarboxylic acid cycle as caused by fluoroacetate (see page 211), and impairment or blockade of the terminal electron transport system as caused by hypoxia or cyanide, all cause abnormal foetal development.

Inhibition of enzymes

Teratogens in this category are also included in some of the previous categories. Enzymes of central importance in intermediary metabolism are particularly vulnerable, such as dihydrofolate reductase, which may be inhibited by folate antagonists giving rise to a deficiency in folic acid. 6-Aminonicotinamide, which inhibits glucose-6-phosphate dehydrogenase, an important enzyme in the pentose-phosphate pathway, is a potent teratogen.

5-Fluorouracil (figure 3.2) an inhibitor of thymidylate synthetase, and cytosine arabinoside, which inhibits DNA polymerase, are both teratogens which have already been referred to.

Changes in osmolarity

Various conditions and agents may change the osmolarity within the developing embryo and thereby disrupt embryogenesis. Thus, induction of hypoxia may cause hypo-osmolarity, which leads to changes in fluid concentrations. This causes changes in pressure and the consequent disruption of tissues may result in abnormal embryogenesis. Other agents causing osmolar changes are hypertonic solutions, certain hormones and compounds such as the azo dye trypan blue, and benzhydryl piperazine. Trypan blue has been widely studied and causes fluid changes in rodent embryos leading to malformations of the brain, eyes, vertebral column and cardiovascular system. It may also have other effects, however, such as inhibition of lysosomal enzymes, which may interfere with release of nutrients from the yolk sac, impairing foetal nutrition.

Benzhydryl piperazine causes orofacial malformations in rat embryos, possibly the result of the oedema induced in the embryo.

Membrane permeability changes

Changes in membrane permeability might be expected to lead to osmolar imbalance and foetal abnormality. This is hypothetical, as there are no real examples of such a mechanism, although high doses of vitamin A are teratogenic and may cause ultrastructural membrane damage.

Transplacental carcinogenesis

Finally, brief mention should be made of the phenomenon of transplacental carcinogenesis. This is the induction of cancer in the offspring by exposure of the pregnant female. It may not occur in the foetus or even in the neonate, but may be evident only in adulthood. The best known example of this is the appearance of vaginal cancer in human females born of mothers given the drug diethylstilboestrol (figure 6.13) during pregnancy. The vaginal cancer did not appear in the female offspring until puberty.

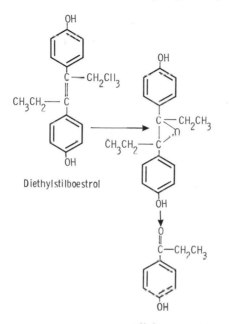

Diethylstilboestrol

p-Hydroxyphenyl ethyl ketone

Figure 6.13. Metabolism of diethylstilboestrol via an epoxide intermediate. This potentially reactive intermediate may show an affinity for the oestradiol receptor and thereby accumulate in oestrogen target organs. This may facilitate reaction with DNA in these organs. From Metzler & McLachlan (1979), *Archs. Toxicol.,* Suppl. 2, 275.

Immunogenesis

Introduction

An immunological or allergic reaction to a foreign compound is a type of toxic response which may be manifested in a variety of ways, and various organ systems may therefore be involved in the response. The skin is commonly involved in man. The severity of the lesion can be minor, such as a small skin rash, or fatal as in the case of anaphylactic shock (see below).

Although the manifestations and severity of an immunological reaction may vary widely with different foreign compounds, there does seem to be a general underlying mechanism. However, the type of response does not depend directly upon the chemical structure of the foreign compound.

Characteristics of immunological reactions

Dose–response relationship

There is generally no clear dose relationship for the production of an immunological reaction. It seems that the magnitude of the response is not determined by the concentration or dose of the foreign compound but by the immunological surveillance mechanism. However, there may sometimes be a rank-order relationship between the occurrence of such an immunological reaction and the total exposure to the foreign compound.

Exposure

Chronic exposure or repeated dosing are required for this type of toxic reaction. Single doses of foreign compounds are not normally immunogenic. Sensitization may occur by repeated or chronic exposure even to very small amounts of the compound such as might occur with environmental exposure. Following sensitization, single doses of minute amounts of the offending substance may be sufficient to elicit a severe response.

Specificity

The nature and extent of the immunological reaction does not generally relate directly to the chemical structure of the compound. Many different compounds, such as *p*-aminobenzoic acid, ethylenediamine and neomycin, cause dermatitis. However, chemically similar compounds may show cross-reactivity: following sensitization by one compound, a chemically very similar compound may, but not always, trigger the same immunological reaction. However, specificity in some cases may be total, this characteristic being utilized in the analytical procedure of immunoassay.

Mechanisms of immunological reactions

The mechanisms underlying immunological reactions are complex and it is beyond the scope of this book to explore them in any depth. It is clear, however, that a general mechanism involves the production of an antibody specific for the antigen or foreign agent (figure 6.14). In the case of most foreign compounds the molecular size is too small for them to function as antigens. However, conjugation of the foreign compound with a protein or other macromolecule may provide the antigen. Although the chemical structure of the foreign compound may determine the reactivity towards suitable macromolecules, it is the nature of the antigenic product which determines the response. Toxic foreign compounds of large molecular size, such as bacterial toxins produced by other organisms, may elicit an immunological reaction in their own right.

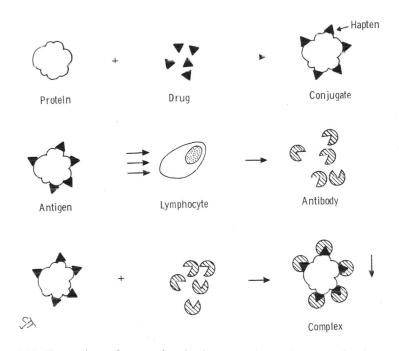

Figure 6.14. Formation of an antigenic drug–protein conjugate and subsequent stimulation of antibody production. The antibody so produced combines with the conjugate and inactivates it, in some cases by causing precipitation of the complex.

The production of an antigen is usually the result of a covalent interaction between the toxic substance and a host protein, and is followed by the synthesis of an antibody. This antibody, a large, complex protein molecule, is specific for the antigen in question and combines with it. This combination may be recognized experimentally as precipitation (precipitin reaction).

Antibodies are known to be proteins, the immunoglobulins IgA, IgG, IgM, IgD and IgE. They have certain common structural features, particularly the heavy and light polypeptide chains, which have certain regions of constant structure and others of variable structure. The variable region varies in its amino acid content, although the number of amino acid residues remains constant. This basic structure is found in almost all animal species.

The antibody is structurally symmetrical and has binding sites for antigens on the variable sections of both light and heavy chains. Antibodies are produced by the lymphoid cells, which are capable of producing large amounts of specific antibodies, one from each cell group. The lymphoid cells are stimulated to divide and produce antibody by the presence of the antigen and more than one antibody may be produced in response to a single antigen. Some antibodies, such as IgG and IgM, are found in plasma, whereas others, IgE for instance, are associated with cells in other tissues.

An immunological response occurs on formation of an antibody–antigen complex. It may involve complement, a complex cascade-type system of serum proteins, which have various cellular effects, and therefore modify the response. The complement proteins released by the antibody–antigen interaction may damage cell surfaces, causing cell death and lysis, initiate histamine release from mast cells and platelets, increase leukocyte phagocytosis and cause smooth muscle to contract.

The immunological response may be mediated by humoral antibodies, cytotropic antibodies or by lymphoid cells, and can be divided into four types of mechanism.

Reactions mediated by circulating cytotropic antibodies. These cytotropic antibodies, such as IgE, become fixed to the cell surface in certain tissues, and when so attached may bind the antigen. This causes the release of compounds such as histamine, serotonin and heparin.

Reactions mediated by serum antibodies against target cells. The antibody complexes with antigens attached to the surface of target cells such as leucocytes, erythrocytes or platelets. The complex causes agglutination or lysis if complement is released.

Reactions involving circulating antigens. Soluble antibody–antigen complexes are formed, giving rise to tissue damage in blood vessels when complement is present.

Reactions mediated by sensitized lymphocytes. In this type of immunological response, the interaction between the antigen and sensitized lymphocytes results in tissue injury.

It is clear that the final response will be determined by the type of antibody involved. With most foreign compounds, apart from proteins or other macromolecules of biological origin, molecular size is insufficient for antigenicity. Small foreign molecules are termed haptens and require conjugation with endogenous protein for antigenic activity. Synthetic hapten–protein conjugates may also be prepared for experimental studies. In some cases it has been shown that the antibody is highly specific for the hapten molecule. Slight changes in structure, such as movement of an amino group from the *o*- to *p*-position on a benzene ring may be sufficient to remove immunogenicity.

The manifestations *in vivo* of an immunological or allergic response may be localized or widespread, immediate or delayed. There may be a localized skin reaction involving an area of only a few square centimetres or a full-blown life-threatening anaphylactic response involving the whole body.

Examples of immediate responses to an immunogenic stimulus are smooth muscle spasms, mucous-membrane oedema and vascular damage. The target organs are generally the skin, blood vessels and the respiratory and gastrointestinal tracts. Anaphylaxis, probably the most serious immunological reaction, is a type I reaction which results from cytotropic antibodies (reagins) such as IgE. Such antibodies circulate in the blood but have a high affinity for the surface of mast cells. The antigen interacts with the mast cell and IgE, giving rise to a reaction. This reaction may entail release of histamine, serotonin, kinins, heparin and slow-reacting substances of anaphylaxis (SRSA). IgG and IgM antibodies (blocking antibodies) may combine with the antigen and inactivate it before it reaches the IgE. The effects of an anaphylactic reaction are difficulty in breathing, loss of blood pressure, anoxia, oedema of the respiratory tract and bronchospasm which may terminate in death. Another manifestation is the serum sickness syndrome which results from IgG antibodies with complement involvement and which consists of arthralgia, fever, lymphadenopathy and sometimes urticaria. Dermatitis may sometimes be a delayed manifestation of an immunological response. This can be widespread or localized and may result from dermal contact with the compound or after administration by various routes. Histamine is probably involved in this type of reaction. Immunological reactions may also lead to serious effects such as anaemia due to the destruction of blood cells. This may result from lysis of the blood cells, which occurs when complement is involved in the immunological response, or by removal of blood cells in the spleen if precipitation or agglutination occurs. For instance, administration of the drug aminopyrine may cause granulocytopoenia which results from the agglutination of leucocytes. It seems that some substance is present in the bloodstream of victims which is capable of causing this agglutination of leucocytes when the drug is administered.

Mutagenesis

Introduction

A mutation is a heritable change produced in the cell genotype. Such a change may be induced by a variety of agents, including foreign compounds, and its occurrence implies that the DNA double helical molecule, the source of genetic information, has been changed.

The genetic code incorporated in this DNA molecule consists of pairs of bases arranged in triplets. The bases utilized are the purine bases adenine (A) and guanine (G), and the pyrimidine bases, thymine (T) and cytosine (C). The basic mechanism of the transfer of the information encoded in DNA is shown in figure 6.15. The information in the DNA molecule may be *replicated* in another identical molecule, *transcribed* into RNA and *translated* into protein.

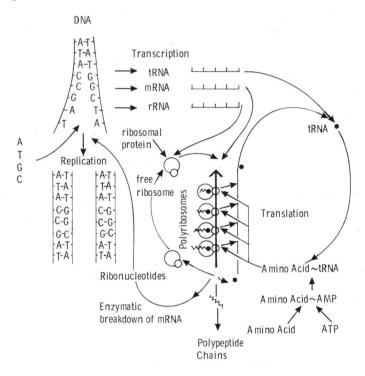

Figure 6.15. Replication of DNA and the transcription and translation of its encoded information into RNA and thence protein. Modified from Watson, J. D. (1965) *The Molecular Biology of the Gene* (New York: W. A. Benjamin).

The three-base code may specify an amino acid in the protein for which the particular gene is responsible or it may specify an instruction such as start or stop translating the code. The DNA molecule, the double helix, is replicated at cell division, during mitosis, for passage to the daughter cells and during meiosis in germ cells for passage to the next generation. This replication is made possible and takes place readily as a result of the base-pairing arrangement within the DNA molecule. The consequence of this specific base pairing is a complementary code on each strand of the molecule, with a purine always paired with a pyrimidine.

Unwinding of the double helical DNA molecule allows each strand to act as a template for new synthesis and guarantees the accurate transmission of information. Alteration of the DNA molecule, in particular a change in the base code, may therefore result in a mutation, although this is not always the result. Such alterations in the base code are of various kinds, each having particular consequences, as described below.

Base-pair transformations. In this type of change, a base, either a purine or a pyrimidine, may be replaced by another. If the replacement base is of the same type, i.e., if a purine is replaced by another purine, this is known as a base-pair transition. If a purine replaces a pyrimidine this is known as a base-pair transversion.

Base-pair addition or deletion. The complete removal or incorporation of a base-pair is more serious than the foregoing and may result in a frameshift mutation. Here the order of the genetic code is altered and hence the reading from that base code is shifted.

Large deletions and rearrangements. Breakage of the complete DNA molecule may occur at one or more sites. This may then be followed by reconstitution of the molecule. One result of this may be erroneous reconstitution, leading to a large change in the genetic code. This type of mutation may also occur at the level of the chromosome when segments may become inverted.

Unequal partition or non-disjunction. The unequal division of chromosomes during mitosis may sometimes occur. This may be the result of exposure of the cell to agents which damage or disturb the spindle fibres or interfere in some way with the process of cell division. The result is a cell with more or less chromosomes than normal, which may or may not be viable.

Thus there are two types of mutagen: those acting directly on DNA and those acting on the replication or the partition of chromosomes. Mutagens of the latter type may therefore only be effective at certain times in the cell cycle. Also, some mutagens may not be able to cross the nuclear membrane and are therefore only active at mitosis, when the nuclear material is in the cytoplasm.

Replication of DNA shows great fidelity, due to the repair of errors which occur during the formation of complementary DNA strands and new DNA molecules. Therefore, many mutations which have occurred in the original molecule and those that occur during the replication process are recognized and corrected. Consequently, fewer mutations are actually present in the replicated DNA molecules than originally occurred. The erroneous bases which are the result of transformations or chemical modification are excised by repair enzymes before the mistake is encoded in the daughter molecule. If the mutation is not recognized and repaired, however, the false information is transcribed into RNA, and hence the error or mutation is expressed as an altered protein resulting from perhaps a single amino acid change. Such a slight change may drastically alter a protein if it occurs at a crucial site in the molecule. For example, in some of the inherited metabolic anaemias this is the case, with a single amino acid change in the haemoglobin molecule being sufficient to drastically impair its function. However, it is clear that only mutations recognized as errors will be repaired and therefore not transcribed. A mutation in the DNA molecule, if not recognized, may therefore be transcribed into mRNA, and the wrong amino acid will be specified and hence translated into a mutant protein. This will occur provided the original mutation is compatible with the transfer RNA codes. Alternatively, the protein may be terminated prematurely and be too short and therefore unable to function. The change may be of no consequence or may be crucial, depending on the position of the amino acid(s) in the protein specified by the gene in question. Mutations may of course lead to an improvement in the gene product.

The mutation is passed on to the daughter cells if not recognized at replication. However, if the mutation is simply an altered base at replication, it will be corrected in one half of the molecule but compounded in the other. For a simple mutation, therefore, involving small changes in the code, the consequence will be of variable severity because:

(*a*) The code for amino acids is degenerate. This means that there may be several codes for any one amino acid and consequently a mutation may be hidden and no change in the amino acid will be seen.

(*b*) A change in the code may change an amino acid in an inconsequential position such as in a structural or terminal portion of the protein.

(*c*) There are nonsense codes which do not specify amino acids but specify instructions such as 'start' or 'stop' transcription or translation. A mutation in such a code might therefore have a profound effect. Alternatively, mutations in the base sequence may give rise to such nonsense codes, causing erroneous instructions to be carried out such as the premature termination of a protein. Obviously, mutations of this kind may have a much more profound effect than a single change in an amino acid.

Base-pair transformations

The smallest unit of mutation is the transformation of a single base pair. There are two mechanisms by which this may occur:

(*a*) The chemical modification of a base;

(*b*) The incorporation of a mutagen into the DNA molecule or a mutagen causing erroneous base pairing.

The first type of base-pair transformation may occur at any stage of the cell cycle. An example of such a transformation is the deamination of the bases adenine and cytosine, caused by nitrous acid. Adenine is deaminated to hypoxanthine, cytosine to uracil (figure 6.16).

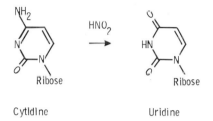

Figure 6.16. Deamination of cytidine to uridine by the action of nitrous acid.

For instance, if such a transformation is induced in the tobacco mosaic virus genome, changes in the viral protein can be detected which correlate with the mutation. This has been made possible because the viral protein has been characterized. Thus it is found that the amino acid threonine is replaced by isoleucine. It is also clear that several triplet codes in the nucleic acid specify the amino acid threonine, namely ACA, AGG, ACC and ACU, emphasizing the degeneracy of the code.

Changing the cytosine to uracil, such as by deamination, in these codes gives AUC, AUA and AUU, the codes which specify isoleucine. This mutation is therefore a C→U transition. The effect of a base-pair transformation on replicating DNA can be seen in figure 6.17, using the example of the deamination of adenine to hypoxanthine which results in a mutagenic transition of the type A : T →G : C. It can be seen that only one of the product DNA molecules has the altered base pair, GC, and therefore only one of the daughter cells is affected. However, this may not necessarily be the case, as some experimental evidence suggests that before replication the partner of the abnormal base may be excised and replaced. Therefore, both strands of the molecule will contain the mutagenic transition.

The expression of the mutant genotype depends in turn on certain factors such as the turnover rate of the product proteins, the rapidity of cell division and, in diploid organisms, the dominance or recessivity of the mutation.

Similar types of mutation are caused by mutagens which alkylate bases, such as the alkyl nitrosamines, which alkylate the N^7 and O^6 of guanine (figure 6.2). This may lead to a G : C→A : T transition.

The second type of base-pair transformation, incorporation of an abnormal base analogue, only occurs at replication of the DNA molecule. An example

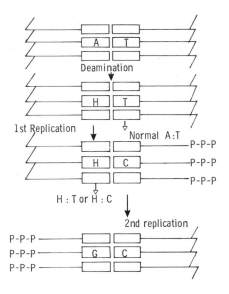

Figure 6.17. Mechanism of a mutagenic transformation by deamination of adenine to hypoxanthine. Hypoxanthine (figure 4.29) pairs like guanine and this results in a transition A : T→G : C. Adapted from Goldstein *et al.* (1974) *Principles of Drug Action: The Basis of Pharmacology* (New York: John Wiley).

of such a mutagen is the thymine analogue, 5-bromouracil (Bu). This compound is incorporated extensively into the DNA molecule during replication, being inserted opposite adenine in place of thymine. 5-bromouracil first forms the deoxyribose triphosphate derivative, a prerequisite for incorporation. If 5-bromouracil is incorporated opposite A, it seems that the A : Bu pair will function as A : T, and the organism continues to grow and divide. Therefore, this change does not seriously affect the function of the DNA. Bu may pair with G, however, as if it were C (figure 6.18), with the consequence that G : C→A : T and A : T→G : C transitions result. The first type of transition occurs because of erroneous incorporation, the second results from erroneous replication against the incorporated Bu. Other base analogues, some of which are used as anti-cancer drugs, may produce lethal mutations in mammalian cells, particularly in cancerous cells which are involved in rapid DNA synthesis.

Frameshift mutations

This type of mutation arises from the addition or deletion of a base to the nucleic acid molecule. This puts the triplet code of the genome out of sequence. Consequently, transcription of the information is erroneous when it is

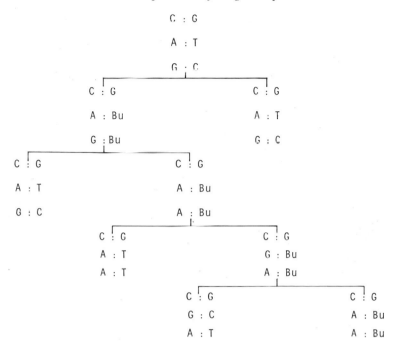

Figure 6.18. Replication of a nucleic acid in the presence of the base analogue bromouracil (Bu). After the first replication, Bu enters opposite guanine (G), giving a G:C→A:T transition. If G enters opposite Bu already incorporated, an A:T→G:C transition results. Adapted from Goldstein *et al.* (1974) *Principles of Drug Action: The Basis of Pharmacology* (New York: John Wiley).

carried out distal to the mutant addition or deletion. In illustration of this, the following code makes sense when read in groups of three:

HOW CAN THE RAT EAT

After the deletion or insertion of a base, however, the code makes no sense:

HOW CAN THR ATE AT...

The transcription of information is therefore generally seriously affected by a frameshift mutation, as large parts of the code may be out of register:

ACA	AAG	AGU	CCA	UCA
threonine	lysine	serine	provaline	serine

becomes

ACA	AGA	GUC	CAU
threonine	lysine	valine	histidine

It is clear that in a long-chain protein produced from such a template, substantial errors may occur.

However, if the addition of a base is followed by a deletion in close proximity or vice versa, production of proteins with partial function may occur.

Frameshift mutations may be produced by various mechanisms. For instance, intercalation of planar molecules, such as acridine within the DNA molecule, allows base insertions at replication. Acridine-type compounds may also induce mutations of the frameshift type by interfering with the excision and repair processes which correct errors occurring during unequal crossover between homologous chromosomes at meiosis. Such unequal crossover gives rise to errors of the frameshift type.

Crossover, which involves the exchange of homologous segments between chromatids at meiosis and between homologous chromatids at mitosis, occurs normally in diploid organisms, by the breaking and reunion of chromatids or by switching of the replication process, a mechanism known as copy choice (figure 6.19). The broken ends of the chromatids which are formed during this process tend to reunite with other broken ends. Any disruption to this system may therefore potentially cause a frameshift mutation. Also, gross alterations of chromosome structure and the complete loss of sections of DNA may occur if the broken section is not attached to the centromere and the chromatids do not move properly at meiosis.

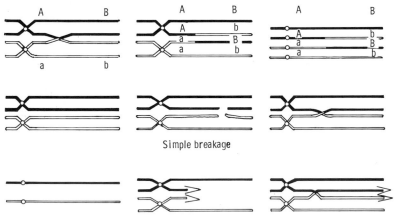

Figure 6.19. Crossover at meiosis. Two homologous chromosomes are shown aligned in the top line. Each consists of two chromatids, joined together at the centromere. A and B represent genes on one chromosome, and a and b the corresponding alleles on the other chromosome. After recombination two new gene combinations are apparent. The middle and bottom lines represent other possible methods of recombination. Adapted from Srb *et al.* (1965) *General Genetics* (San Francisco: W. H. Freeman), after Goldstein *et al.* (1974) *Principles of Drug Action: The Basis of Pharmacology* (New York: John Wiley).

Chromosome breakage and deletions

This type of mutagenic effect is similar to the foregoing but on a larger scale. Certain compounds cause the breakage of chromosomes, including many of those able to induce base-pair transformations. Alkylating agents, both monofunctional and difunctional, cause chromosome breakage, the latter type probably by causing crosslinking across the DNA molecule. Inhibition of DNA repair may be another cause of this type of mutation.

Chromosome breakage may therefore be linked to other mechanisms of mutagenesis in some fundamental manner. The correction of errors involves breakage of the DNA molecule for both the 'cut and patch' type of repair and for sister strand exchange (figure 6.20). Interference with these processes could clearly result in breakage in one or both chains of the DNA molecule, which it is now accepted forms the backbone of the chromatid. Large deletions may also occur after breakage of the chromosome if the repair processes are compromised.

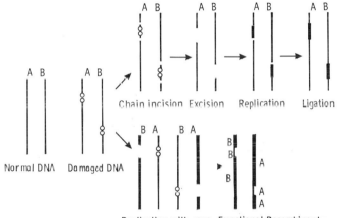

Figure 6.20. Representation of two mechanisms of repair of DNA damage such as ultraviolet light-induced dimerization. The upper line represents cut and patch repair, the lower sister strand exchange. Thick lines represent newly synthesized DNA. Adapted from Goldstein *et al.* (1974) *Principles of Drug Action: The Basis of Pharmacology* (New York: John Wiley).

Metaphase poisoning

This type of mutation involves interference with the processes of mitosis and meiosis. During mitosis, sister chromosomes partition prior to separation of the daughter cells and in meiosis this occurs with homologous chromosomes. The partitioning of chromosomes during these processes requires positioning of the centrioles, then arrangement of the chromosomes in the correct positions at metaphase, formation of spindle fibres and involvement of these in the partition of the chromosomes. Interference with one or more aspects of this overall process constitutes metaphase poisoning.

The spindle fibres are attached to the chromosomes at the centromere and align them on the equatorial plate. The spindle arrangement contains microtubules composed of the protein tubulin. Colchicine is a specific spindle poison, which binds to tubulin, and inhibits its polymerization. Consequently, colchicine blocks mitosis, causing polyploidy, the unequal partition of chromosomes and metaphase arrest.

Other compounds causing such effects are podophyllotoxin and the vinca alkaloids, vincristine and vinblastine.

The unequal partition of chromosomes, or non-disjunction, is a serious effect if the affected daughter cells survive. Down's syndrome or Trisomy 21 is the result of chromosome non-disjunction in man, there being 47 chromosomes instead of 46. This unequal partitioning of chromosomes can occur at mitosis in germ cells or during meiosis in the production of sperm or ova.

Mutagenesis in mammals

The effects of mutagens on mammalian cells *in vivo* are less clearly defined than their effects on bacterial cells. When mutagens act on mammalian germ cells, inherited defects may arise, and when somatic cells are exposed to mutagens, cellular organization may be disrupted, giving rise to tumours. It now seems clear that many mutagens are carcinogens and most if not all carcinogens are mutagenic.

Major mutagenic changes in somatic cells will clearly lead to total disruption of DNA-directed cellular organization, possibly cell death but probably an inability to grow and divide.

Mutagenic attack in rapidly dividing cells, such as in embryonic tissue, will obviously be particularly serious, giving rise to defects in growth and differentiation, leading to birth defects. Consequently, mutagens are often also teratogens, although some are directly cytotoxic, and it may be this rather than their mutagenicity which causes the teratogenic effect.

However, both carcinogenesis and teratogenesis are discussed separately, and therefore attention will be confined to the susceptibility of the germ cell line.

In the human, the primordial germ cells are differentiated from about the sixth week of gestation and are consequently susceptible from then onwards. In the female, production of the primary oocytes, which involves the first meiotic division, occurs in foetal life. These primary oocytes do not mature into ova until puberty, with the second meiotic division yielding one ovum from each primary oocyte (figure 6.21).

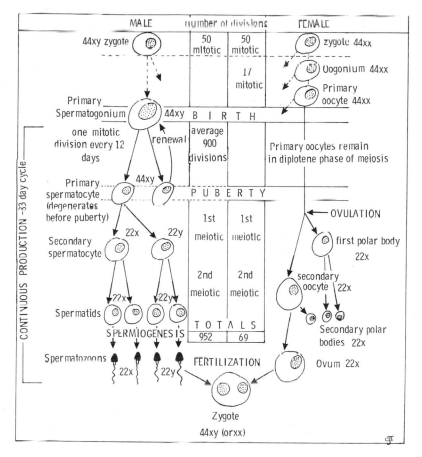

Figure 6.21. Gametogenesis in humans showing the number of nuclear divisions giving rise to the gametes. Each *average* fertilizing spermatozoon is the result of 900 divisions of the primary spermatogonium.

In the male, the stem cells or primary spermatogonia undergo mitotic division regularly, one of the products becoming the primary spermatocyte which, after two meiotic divisions, gives rise to four spermatozoa. This continues throughout childhood, but before puberty the sperms degenerate. In the female organism, chromosomes replicate about 70 times in the production of an ovum while in the male 950 replications take place in the production of a sperm. In both cases, however, only two continuous meiotic divisions have occurred, involving one possible crossover of chromatids.

It is therefore clear that susceptibility to the action of mutagens on the mammalian germ line is different in the female and the male. In the female, mutagens which act on replicating DNA or on the process of mitosis have effects on the foetal germ tissue and possibly on meiosis occurring at maturation of the ovum. Mutagens which act on non-replicating DNA are clearly active throughout the lifetime of the female organism. As the greatest number of mitoses take place in the foetus, exposure to mutagens should be particularly avoided during this time, the first trimester of pregnancy. This is also the period of greatest teratogenic susceptibility. In testing for muta-genic effects in the female mammalian organism, therefore, continuous exposure of the animal to the mutagen may be important, particularly with mutagens which act at the meiosis which occurs during the short period of the maturation of the ovum.

In the male, mutagens which act on replicating DNA or on the process of mitosis do so in the foetus and during the period of reproductive life. Mutagens acting on non-replicating DNA are also active throughout foetal and reproductive life. Agents which are mutagenic at meiosis will be so during the period of maturation of the spermocytes to produce sperm.

As would be predicted, there are large differences in mutagenicity de-pending upon the time of treatment. This reflects the sensitivity of the various stages of spermatogenesis or oogenesis. Therefore, the time after maturation when the organism is exposed to the mutagen and affected by it may give some indication of which stage is sensitive.

Determination of mutagenicity and its relation to carcinogenicity

The potential mutagenicity of a foreign compound may now be rapidly and easily determined using a variety of short-term tests, one of the best known being the Ames test. This test utilizes histidine-requiring mutant strains of *Salmonella* bacteria. If a foreign compound causes a mutation, the bacteria may then grow on histidine-free medium and can be readily detected. The test has been adapted to utilize liver homogenate, usually from rats or other experimental animals, so as to identify mutagens which require metabolic activation (see Bibliography).

As discussed in the preceding section, there is a relationship between mutagenesis and carcinogenesis and the Ames technique is used to predict potential carcinogens. However, although it is clear that many mutagens, as detected in the Ames test, are also carcinogens, there are discrepancies. There are some mutagens which are not carcinogens and some substances shown to be carcinogenic in animals which are not mutagenic. This area of research is controversial and very active.

The test is set up to be extremely sensitive to mutagenic activity and the incorporation of the liver homogenate allows for metabolically activated mutagens. However, the major route of metabolism of a mutagen *in vivo* may be detoxication rather than activation, which may account for some of the false positives, and tumour induction almost certainly requires the occurrence of more events than a mutation, as discussed in the section on carcinogenicity. Consequently, the results of short-term mutagenicity tests must be interpreted with caution as regards potential carcinogenicity.

Miscellaneous toxic effects

Although the liver and kidney are perhaps the organs most commonly associated with tissue damage from toxic compounds, all the other organ systems are also vulnerable. There are examples of compounds which selectively damage certain types of tissue or certain organs. Although it is not within the scope of this book to explore all these in depth, brief mention can be made of some of them to indicate the various types of toxicity which may occur. Of particular interest in toxicology is neurotoxicity, as the nervous system is a common target for the toxic effects of a number of foreign compounds which lead to the development of peripheral neuropathy. Some of the cholinesterase inhibitors are particularly active in this respect, and so is methyl mercury, which is infamous because of its association with Minnamata disease (see page 227). The central nervous system is obviously a highly complex network of specialized cells, and destruction of sections of this system may have prolonged effects on the function of the organism which will probably be permanent, as nerve cells do not regenerate. The cells of the nervous system are particularly sensitive to changes in their environment which may be caused by toxic compounds. Anoxia, restriction of blood flow, lack of glucose and other essential metabolites, and inhibition of intermediary metabolism may all cause damage to nerve cells, and direct damage may be caused by cytotoxic agents.

Another important toxic response is damage to the blood cells, either those circulating or those in the bone marrow. Bone marrow cells are very sensitive to toxic compounds, as they are actively dividing. Damage to the bone marrow may result in reduced numbers of red and/or white blood cells, such as that caused by the solvent benzene (figure 4.3), which produces bone marrow aplasia. Damage to circulating blood cells may also be caused by toxic compounds impairing the oxygen-carrying capacity by interference with haemoglobin, or by actually destroying the red cells by haemolysis as in the case of phenylhydrazine toxicity.

Aromatic amines and amides, including drugs such as phenacetin (figure 5.13), may cause methaemoglobinaemia, the reversible oxidation of haemoglobin, which impairs the oxygen-carrying ability of the red cells. Irreversible damage to haemoglobin may occur as a result of oxidation of thiol groups in the protein, with subsequent denaturation impairment of membrane function and haemolysis of the red cell.

The gonads may be particularly susceptible to the effects of toxic compounds, being prime targets for mutagens as well as cytotoxic agents. The actively dividing tissue in the mature male and in the female during the oestrous cycle is vulnerable to cytotoxic and mutagenic agents which may be transported there. Mutagenic effects will be expressed in the succeeding generations as lethal mutations or malformations *in utero* in the adult animal, but cytotoxic effects may be expressed as decreased fertility and decreased libido. The pesticide dibromochloropropane was found to cause damage to the testis in the male rat, and in humans to lead to infertility. This compound is also a mutagen and a carcinogen. In the female, menstrual disorders may also result from damage to germ cell tissue, such as that caused occasionally by carbon disulphide, which also causes reduced fertility and spontaneous abortions.

Other organs may be selectively damaged, such as the eyes in practolol toxicity (see Chapter 7). Parts of the inner ear may be damaged by antibiotics such as streptomycin, in the pancreas the β-cells may be selectively destroyed by alloxan and streptozoticin, and in the heart cardiomyopathy is thought to be caused by the metal cobalt.

Bibliography

Carcinogenesis

BOYLAND, E. (1980) History and future of chemical carcinogenesis. In Chemical Carcinogenesis, edited by P. Brookes. *British Medical Bulletin*, **36,** 5.

GOLDSTEIN, A., ARONOW, L. & MALMAN, S. M. (1974) *Principles of Drug Action: The Basis of Pharmacology*, Chapter 11 (New York: John Wiley).

LAWLEY, P. D. (1980) DNA as a target of alkylating carcinogens. In Chemical Carcinogenesis, edited by P. Brookes, *British Medical Bulletin*, **36,** 19.

MILLER, E. C. & MILLER, J. A. (1976) The metabolism of chemical carcinogens to reactive electrophiles and their possible mechanism of action in carcinogenesis. In *Chemical Carcinogens*, edited by C. E. Searle (Washington D.C.: American Chemical Society).

SIMS, P. (1980) Metabolic activation of chemical carcinogens. In Chemical Carcinogenesis, edited by P. Brookes, *British Medical Bulletin*, **36,** 11.

WIESBURGER, J. H. & WILLIAMS, G. M. (1980) Chemical carcinogens. In *Casarett and Doull's Toxicology, The Basic Science of Poisons*, edited by J. Doull, C. D. Klaassen and M. O. Amdur (New York: Macmillan).

WILLIAMS, G. M. (1980) The pathogenesis of rat liver cancer caused by chemical carcinogenesis. *Biochim. biophys. Acta*, **605,** 167.

Tissue lesions

BUS, J. S. & GIBSON, J. E. (1979) Lipid peroxidation and its role in toxicology. In *Reviews in Biochemical Toxicology*, Vol. 1, edited by E. Hodgson, J. R. Bend and R. M. Philpot (New York: Elsevier-North Holland).

DAVIS, M., VERGANI, D., MIELI-VERGANI, G., EDDLESTON, A. L. W. F., NEUBERGER, I. M. & WILLIAMS, R. (1981) Immunological studies on the pathogenesis of halothane associated hepatitis. In *Drug Reactions and the Liver*, p. 237, edited by M. Davis, J. M. Tredger and R. Williams (London: Pitman Medical)

HOOK, J. B. (1980) Toxic responses of the kidney. In *Casarett and Doull's Toxicology, The Basic Sciences of Poisons*, edited by J. Doull, C. D. Klaassen and M. O. Amdur (New York: Macmillan).

HOOK, J. B., McCORMACK, K. M. & KLUWE, W. M. (1979) Biochemical mechanisms of nephrotoxicity. In *Reviews in Biochemical Toxicology*, Vol. 1, edited by E. Hodgson, J. R. Bend and R. M. Philpot (New York: Elsevier-North Holland).

KULKARNI, A. P. & HODGSON, E. (1980) Hepatotoxicity. In *Introduction to Biochemical Toxicology*, edited by E. Hodgson and F. E. Guthrie (New York: Elsevier North Holland).

MENZEL, D. B. & McCLELLAN, R. O. (1980) Toxic responses of the respiratory system. In *Casarett and Doull's Toxicology, The Basic Science of Poisons*, edited by J. Doull, C. D. Klaassen and M. O. Amdur (New York: Macmillan).

PLAA, G. L. (1980) Toxic responses of the liver. In *Casarett and Doull's Toxicology, The Basic Science of Poisons*, edited by J. Doull, C. D. Klaassen and M. O. Amdur (New York: Macmillan).

RAPPAPORT, A. M. (1976) The microcirculatory acinar concept of normal and pathological hepatic structure. *Beitr. Path.*, **157**, 215.

SLATER, T. F. (editor) (1978) *Biochemical Mechanisms of Liver Injury* (London: Academic Press).

SMUCKLER, E. A. (1976) Structural and functional changes in acute liver injury. *Environ. Health Perspect.*, **15**, 13.

TRUMP, B. F. & ARSTILA, A. V. (1980) Cellular reaction to injury. In *Principles of Pathobiology*, edited by M. F. La Via and R. B. Hill (New York: Oxford University Press).

ZIMMERMAN, H. J. (1978) *Hepatotoxicity* (New York: Appleton Century Crofts).

Physiological or pharmacological effects

GOLDSTEIN, A., ARONOW, L. & KALMAN, S. M. (1974) *Principles of Drug Action: The Basis of Pharmacology*, Chapter 1, Molecular mechanisms of drug action, and Chapter 5, Drug toxicity (New York: John Wiley).

GOODMAN GILMAN, A., GOODMAN, L. S. & GILMAN, A. (editors) (1980) *Goodman and Gilman's The Pharmacological Basis of Therapeutics* (New York: Macmillan).

Teratogenesis

GOLDSTEIN, A., ARONOW, L. & KALMAN, S. M. (1974) *Principles of Drug Action: The Basis of Pharmacology*, Chapter 12, Chemical teratogenesis (New York: John Wiley).

HARBISON, R D. (1980) Teratogens. In *Casarett and Doull's Toxicology, The Basic Science of Poisons*, edited by J. Doull, C. D. Klaassen and M. O. Amdur (New York: Macmillan).
SULLIVAN, F. M. & BARLOW, S. M. (1979) Congenital malformations and other reproductive hazards from environmental chemicals. *Proc. Roy. Soc. Lond.*, B, **205**, 91.
WILSON, J. G. (1973) *Environment and Birth Defects* (New York: Academic Press).
WILSON, J. G. & FRASER, F. C. (editors) (1977) *Handbook of Teratology*, Vols. 1–4 (New York: Plenum Press).

Immunogenesis

GOLDSTEIN, A., ARONOW, L. & KALMAN, S. M. (1974) *Principles of Drug Action: The Basis of Pharmacology*, Chapter 7, Drug allergy (New York: John Wiley).
ROITT, I. M. (1977) *Essential Immunology* (Oxford: Blackwell Scientific Publications).

Mutagenesis

AMES, B. N. (1979) Identifying environmental chemicals causing mutations and cancer. *Science*, **204**, 587.
DIXON, R. L. (1980) Toxic responses of the reproductive system. In *Casarett and Doull's Toxicology, The Basic Science of Poisons*, edited by J. Doull, C. D. Klaassen and M. O. Amdur (New York: Macmillan).
DRAKE, J. W. (1970) *The Molecular Basis of Mutation* (San Francisco: Holden Day).
GOLDSTEIN, A., ARONOW, L. & KALMAN, S. M. (1974) *Principles of Drug Action: The Basis of Pharmacology*, Chapter 10, Chemical mutagenesis (New York: John Wiley).
GROSCH, D. S. (1980) Genetic Poisons. In *Introduction to Biochemical Toxicology*, edited by E. Hodgson and F. E. Guthrie (New York: Elsevier-North Holland).
HOLLEANDER, A. (editor) (1971–1981) *Chemical Mutagens: Principles and Methods for Their Detection*, several volumes (New York: Plenum Press).
THILLY, W. G. & LIBER, H. L. (1980) Genetic Toxicology. In *Casarett and Doull's Toxicology, The Basic Science of Poisons*, edited by J. Doull, C. D. Klaassen and M. O. Amdur (New York: Macmillan).
VOGEL, F. & ROHRBORN, G. (editors) (1970) *Chemical Mutagenesis in Mammals and Man* (New York: Springer Verlag).

Miscellaneous toxic effects

DOULL, J., KLAASSEN, C. D. & AMDUR, M. O. (editors) (1980) *Casarett and Doull's Toxicology, The Basic Science of Poisons* (New York: Macmillan).
GOLDSTEIN, A., ARONOW, L. & KALMAN, S. M. (1974) *Principles of Drug Action: The Basis of Pharmacology*, Chapter 5, Drug Toxicity (New York: John Wiley).
GORROD, J. W. (editor) (1979) *Drug Toxicity* (London: Taylor & Francis).
HODGSON, E. & GUTHRIE, F. E. (editors) (1980) *Introduction to Biochemical Toxicology* (New York: Elsevier-North Holland).

Chapter 7

Biochemical mechanisms of toxicity: specific examples

Chemical carcinogenesis

Acetylaminofluorene

This compound is a well known carcinogen and one of the most widely studied. Research into the mechanism underlying its carcinogenicity is at present an area of high activity and therefore this discussion must confine itself to the principles rather than details.

The study of acetylaminofluorene carcinogenicity has provided insight into the carcinogenicity of other aromatic amines and also illustrates a number of other important points. Acetylaminofluorene is a very potent mutagen and a carcinogen in a number of animal species, causing tumours primarily of the liver, bladder and the kidney. It became clear from research that metabolism of the compound was involved in the carcinogenicity. The important metabolic reaction was found to be N-hydroxylation, catalysed by the microsomal mixed function oxidases, and this was demonstrated both *in vitro* and *in vivo*. Thus N-hydroxyacetylaminofluorene (figure 7.1), the product, is a more potent carcinogen than the parent compound. The production of this metabolite *in vivo* was found to be increased nine-fold by the repeated administration of the parent compound, a finding of particular importance when considering the general use of single-dose rather than multiple low-dose studies for evaluating the toxicity of compounds. This effect is presumably the result of induction of the microsomal enzymes involved in the production of N-hydroxyacetylaminofluorene. N-hydroxylation has since proved to be an important metabolic reaction in the toxicity of a number of other compounds. The N-hydroxy intermediate in particular

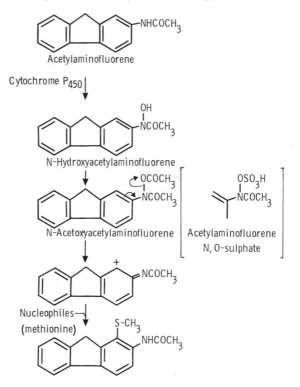

Figure 7.1. Metabolic activation of acetylaminofluorene. Formation of the *N,O*-acetate or *N,O*-sulphate of *N*-hydroxyacetylaminofluorene is followed by the production of a reactive carbonium ion intermediate which reacts with nucleophiles such as methionine. The products of this reaction have been isolated and include 3-methylmercapto-2-acetylaminofluorene.

is of importance for the carcinogenicity of a number of aromatic amino, nitro and nitroso compounds. This intermediate may arise by reduction as well as oxidation (see page 66). However, *N*-hydroxyacetylaminofluorene is not the ultimate carcinogen, as it requires further metabolism in order to initiate tumour production. The *N*-hydroxylated intermediate is stable enough to be conjugated and the N-O glucuronide of acetylaminofluorene is an important metabolite (figure 4.47).

It was found that some conjugates of *N*-hydroxyacetylaminofluorene were more potent carcinogens than the parent compound or its *N*-hydroxy metabolite. Thus the acetate ester, acetoxyacetylaminofluorene, is one such potent carcinogen which was found to react with the amino acid methionine *in vitro*. The product of this reaction, isolated after the work-up procedure, was 3-methylmercaptoacetylaminofluorene, the same as isolated from tissues *in vivo* after treatment with acetylaminofluorene (figure 7.1). Acetoxyacetyl-aminofluorene also reacts with the nucleoside guanosine monophosphate, to yield 8-guanylacetylaminofluorene *in vitro*. This conjugate has also been detected in studies *in vivo*. There are various routes of formation for the acetoxy derivative, such as enzymically via an acetyl transferase or by transacetylation. The alkylation of DNA and nuclear proteins by acetyl-aminofluorene has also been demonstrated.

Another N–O conjugate thought to be possibly involved in the carcino-genicity is the N–O sulphate ester (figure 7.1). The formation of this con-jugate, catalysed by a sulphotransferase enzyme and utilizing PAPS (see Chapter 4) takes place in the soluble fraction of the cell. Although acetyla-minofluorene N–O sulphate has low carcinogenicity when applied to the skin of experimental animals, it is an extremely reactive and unstable compound. It seems that the acetoxy and sulphate groups are chemically described as 'good leaving groups', thereby readily producing the reactive carbonium ion postulated to be the reactive intermediate (figure 7.1). The involvement of sulphate conjugation brings other factors into play. Depletion of body sulphate reduces and supplementation with organic sulphate increases the carcinogenicity of acetylaminofluorene. The production of covalent adducts between acetylaminofluorene and cellular macromolecules *in vivo* can be shown to be correspondingly decreased and increased by manipulation of body sulphate levels.

Although the N–O glucuronide has a lower chemical reactivity and carcinogenicity than the sulphate conjugate, the glucuronide may be respon-sible for the production of bladder cancer by acetylaminofluorene. Further-more, the N O sulphate conjugate is not the only ultimate carcinogen, as acetylaminofluorene induces tumours in tissues without sulphotransferase activity. However, the ability of a tissue to conjugate acetylaminofluorene with sulphate does correlate with the carcinogenicity.

N-hydroxylation is not the only or major route of metabolism *in vivo*, nor is it the only reaction catalysed by the microsomal enzymes. Ring hydroxylation is the major route of metabolism, the products of which are not carcinogenic. These alternative routes of metabolism are inducible *in vivo* by pretreatment with agents such as phenobarbital and 3-methylcholanthrene (see Chapter 5). Glucuronidation of the resulting hydroxyl derivatives is also induced by phenobarbital pretreatment. Consequently, pretreatment of animals with both these agents reduces the carcinogenicity of acetylamino-fluorene. This illustrates the difficulty of predicting the effect of environmental influences on toxicity when multiple metabolic pathways are involved.

Another route of metabolism for acetylaminofluorene is deacetylation. Both the parent compound and the metabolite *N*-hydroxyacetylamino-fluorene are deacetylated by hydrolytic enzymes found in both the soluble and microsomal cell fractions. Deacetylation of *N*-hydroxyacetylamino-fluorene is thought to take place in the microsomal fraction.

A well documented species difference in susceptibility to acetylamino-fluorene carcinogenicity is the resistance of the guinea-pig. This affords an interesting illustration of the role of species differences in metabolism as a basis for species differences in susceptibility to toxicity. The guinea-pig is not resistant to the carcinogenicity of the metabolite N-hydroxyacetylamino-fluorene, however, indicating that this species has low activity for N-hydroxylation. As well as this, the guinea-pig has low sulphotransferase activity but a highly active microsomal deacetylase, particularly with N-hydroxyacetylaminofluorene as the substrate. A combination of these three factors therefore confers resistance on the guinea-pig. The low produc-tion of N-hydroxyacetylaminofluorene followed by low sulphate conjugation result in little of the ultimate carcinogen being produced. Furthermore, deacetylation of N-hydroxyacetylaminofluorene to yield N-hydroxyamino-fluorene, which is not carcinogenic, also decreases carcinogenicity.

The study of acetylaminofluorene carcinogenesis therefore provides many insights into the factors affecting chemical carcinogenesis. A wealth of other data not discussed here is available which confirms the occurrence of covalent interactions between the ultimate carcinogenic metabolite of acetylamino-fluorene and nucleic acids to yield covalent conjugates (figure 7.1). It remains to be seen how these conjugates initiate the process of carcinogenesis.

Benzo[a]pyrene

The polycyclic aromatic hydrocarbons constitute a large group of com-pounds, which includes a number of carcinogens found originally in coal tar but which have since been detected in cigarette smoke, the exhaust fumes from internal combustion engines, and smoke from other processes involving the burning of organic material. Benzo[a]pyrene is one of the most intensely studied, as it is an extremely potent carcinogen. Although chemically stable, *in vivo* polycyclic aromatic hydrocarbons undergo a wide variety of metabolic transformations catalysed by the microsomal mixed-function oxidases as illustrated for benzo[a]pyrene (figure 7.2). These are mainly hydroxylations occurring at the various available sites on the aromatic rings, and conjuga-tions of the hydroxyl groups with glucuronic acid or sulphate. The majority of these hydroxylation reactions probably proceed through an epoxide intermediate, as discussed in Chapter 4.

Initially, particular attention was focused on the epoxides of the so-called K region. As in the case of benzo[a]pyrene and certain other polycyclic aromatic hydrocarbons, these were more carcinogenic than the parent compound. The K region had attracted particular interest, as it is electroni-cally the most reactive portion of the polycyclic aromatic hydrocarbon molecule. However, with other carcinogenic polycyclic aromatic hydro-carbons this was not found to be the case. It now seems that the ultimate

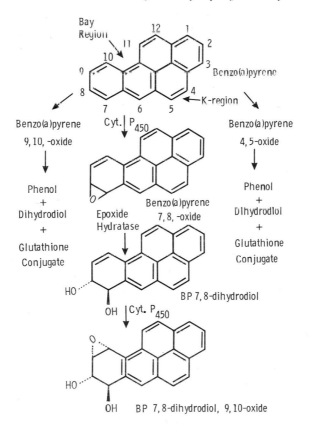

Figure 7.2. Metabolism of benzo[*a*]pyrene. The major sites for hydroxylation are the 4, 5, 7, 8 and 9, 10 positions, giving rise to numerous phenols and their conjugates and also to dihydrodiols and glutathione conjugates. Formation of the epoxide of the 7,8-dihydrodiol is thought to be the crucial step in the carcinogenesis.

carcinogen is an epoxide of a dihydrodiol metabolite where the epoxide is adjacent to the so-called bay region (figure 7.2). It is postulated that this ultimate carcinogen reacts covalently with nucleic acids, producing nucleic acid adducts. It has been demonstrated that benzo[*a*]pyrene reacts covalently with nucleic acids *in vitro*, provided that the microsomal enzyme systems necessary for activation are present, and also in whole cell systems. The 7,8-dihydrodiol metabolite of benzo[*a*]pyrene binds more extensively to DNA after microsomal enzyme activation than does benzo[*a*]pyrene or other benzo[*a*]pyrene metabolites, and the nucleoside adducts formed from the 7,8-dihydrodiol of benzo[*a*]pyrene are similar to those obtained from cells in culture exposed to benzo[*a*]pyrene itself. Furthermore, the synthetic 7,8-diol-9,10-epoxides of benzo[*a*]pyrene are highly mutagenic in mammalian as well as in bacterial cells.

Other studies of DNA adducts formed *in vivo* with benzo[a]pyrene and using cells in culture have also indicated that the 7,8-diol-9,10-epoxides are responsible for most of the covalent binding to nucleic acids, even though the K region, 4,5-epoxide is highly mutagenic. The 7,8-epoxide for benzo[a]pyrene and the 7,8-dihydrodiol are carcinogenic, but the 4,5- and 9,10-epoxides are not. These findings all point towards the conclusion that the further metabolism of the 7,8-epoxide of benzo[a]pyrene by epoxide hydratase to the dihydrodiol metabolite and then further oxidation of the dihydrodiol by the mixed function oxidases to the diol-epoxide are the necessary steps for production of the ultimate carcinogen. These metabolic transformations are illustrated in figure 7.2. Other possible reactive intermediates which have been postulated are radicals and radical cations.

The coplanarity of benzo[a]pyrene and many carcinogenic polycyclic hydrocarbons is of interest. It has been suggested that this flat structure allows intercalation of the hydrocarbon within the DNA molecule, thereby facilitating reaction of the intermediate with the nucleic acid.

It is clear that the effects of induction or inhibition of the metabolism will be complex, due to the large number of possible metabolic pathways through which benzo[a]pyrene may be metabolized. For instance, the microsomal enzyme inducer 5,6-benzoflavone inhibits the carcinogenicity of benzo[a]pyrene to mouse lung and skin, whereas inhibitors such as SKF 525A may increase the tumour production from certain polycyclic hydrocarbons.

Dimethylnitrosamine

Nitrosamines are very potent carcinogens which, *in vivo*, act as alkylating agents. Dimethylnitrosamine is one of the most intensively studied, causing tumours of the liver, kidney and lung in rats and tumours in other species. It is also acutely toxic, single doses causing centrilobular hepatic necrosis, but not hepatic tumours, in adult rats. Metabolic studies have shown that it is distributed evenly throughout the animal body, but only causes damage to, and tumours in, certain organs, indicating that the metabolism of this substance is probably involved in its carcinogenicity. Using radiolabelled dimethylnitrosamine, this was indeed found to be the case.

The structure and metabolism of dimethylnitrosamine are shown in figure 7.3. The metabolism involves initial carbon hydroxylation, catalysed by the microsomal enzymes, followed by the loss of one methyl group as formaldehyde. The intermediate monomethylnitrosamine (figure 7.3) is then thought to rearrange to yield a diazohydroxide, a diazonium ion and finally an alkyl carbonium ion and nitrogen. This alkyl carbonium ion is a highly reactive alkylating agent which may methylate sites on proteins and nucleic acids.

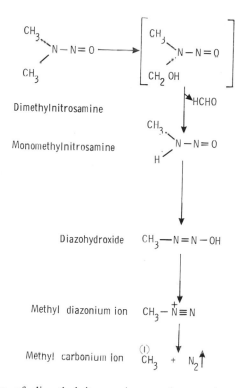

Dimethylnitrosamine

Monomethylnitrosamine

Figure 7.3. Metabolism of dimethylnitrosamine to the reactive carbonium ion intermediate responsible for methylation of nucleic acids and thought to be the ultimate carcinogen.

The acute toxicity is reduced in animals pretreated with the microsomal enzyme inducers 3-methylcholanthrene and phenobarbital, and these pre-treatments also protect animals from the carcinogenic effects. Phenobarbital and 3-methylcholanthrene reduce demethylation. However, inhibition of metabolism by certain compounds also protects animals against the toxic and carcinogenic effects of dimethylnitrosamine. It is therefore clear that there may be several pathways of metabolism, some of which may detoxify dimethylnitrosamine, and hence this may explain the protective effects of microsomal enzyme-inducing agents.

The methylation of various sites in nucleic acids, mainly the N^7 and the O^6 position of guanine, has been readily demonstrated both *in vivo* and *in vitro*. The DNA alkylation reactions carried out by nitrosamines *in vivo* are in fact very similar to those *in vitro*, and the degree of methylation of DNA *in vivo* in different tissues parallels the ability of dimethylnitrosamine to induce tumours in those tissues. It also seems that the ability of a tissue to

G

repair the alkylated bases may be a major factor in its susceptibility to the carcinogen.

The methylation of DNA, however, is greater in the liver than in any other organ, including the kidney, after a single dose of dimethylnitrosamine; yet such single doses rarely cause hepatic tumours, but do induce tumours in the kidney. Therefore, it seems that the liver may initially have greater resistance to the carcinogenicity of dimethylnitrosamine, due to protective mechanisms, but that these may be compromised by repeated doses of the carcinogen, thereby allowing tumour induction in the liver after chronic exposure.

Treatment of neonatal animals, or those subjected to partial hepatectomy, with single doses of dimethylnitrosamine, leads to hepatic tumours, as in these cases the liver cells are actively dividing and are more susceptible. It has been found that the liver cells in culture are susceptible at particular stages in the cell cycle.

The metabolic activity of various tissues is also a determinant of susceptibility to tumour production. The gastrointestinal tract is resistant to dimethylnitrosamine carcinogenesis, even when the compound is given orally, as the metabolic activity of this organ is low as far as activation of dimethylnitrosamine is concerned.

The diet of the animal may also influence organ sensitivity to this carcinogen. For instance, protein-deficient diets reduce the toxicity of the compound but increase the incidence of kidney tumours. A concomittant increase in the methylation of nucleic acids in the kidney is observed under these conditions. It was concluded from this and other evidence that a protein-deficient diet decreased metabolism of dimethylnitrosamine in the liver, but did not decrease it in the kidney, and so this and other organs were exposed to a higher concentration of unchanged carcinogen in the protein-deficient animals.

Tissue lesions: liver necrosis

Carbon tetrachloride

The hepatotoxicity of carbon tetrachloride has probably been more extensively studied than that of any other hepatotoxin, and there is now a wealth of data available. Its toxicity has been studied both from biochemical and pathological viewpoints, and therefore provides many insights into mechanisms of toxicity.

Carbon tetrachloride is a simple molecule which, when administered to a variety of species, causes centrilobular hepatic necrosis and fatty liver. It is very lipid-soluble and is consequently well distributed throughout the body, but despite this its major toxic effect is on the liver, irrespective of the route of administration. Low doses of carbon tetrachloride cause only fatty liver and destruction of hepatic cytochrome P-450. However, chronic administration or exposure leads to liver cirrhosis, in some instances liver cancer and also kidney damage.

Although originally thought to be resistant to metabolic attack it is now known to be metabolized by the microsomal enzymes, almost certainly via a free radical. The hepatotoxicity of carbon tetrachloride is increased by microsomal enzyme inducers and decreased by inhibitors, indicating that metabolic activation is required for hepatotoxicity. The production of necrosis, particularly in the centrilobular region, is probably the result of the higher levels of cytochrome P-450 in this region, although the absence or lower level of protective mechanisms may be another factor. The postulated metabolic activation is shown in figure 7.4.

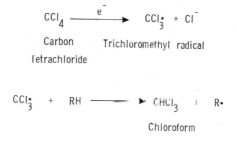

Figure 7.4. Microsomal enzyme-mediated metabolic activation of carbon tetrachloride. The trichloromethyl radical so produced may take a hydrogen atom from a suitable donor to yield chloroform and a secondary radical.

The role of the microsomal enzymes is therefore as an electron donor. The trichloromethyl radical so produced may then react in a variety of ways with cellular constituents. Abstraction of a hydrogen atom leads to the production of chloroform, an observed metabolite (figure 7.4). Chloroform is produced in microsomes *in vitro* in the absence of air, indicating that the metabolic transformation, although dependent upon cytochrome P-450, probably involves some form of electron transfer, independent of oxygen. The trichloromethyl radical is reactive, although recent work indicates that it may not be sufficiently reactive, and the trichloromethyl peroxy radical ($CCl_3O_2\cdot$) has been postulated as an alternative by Slater (1980). Whatever the reactive intermediate produced, it will have a small radius of action. The immediate damage caused by the carbon tetrachloride is therefore in the smooth endoplasmic reticulum, the site of metabolic activation, and cytochrome P-450 is destroyed. This destruction, which can be studied *in vitro*, requires oxygen.

Small doses of carbon tetrachloride destroy hepatic cytochrome P-450, decreasing activity *in vivo* by 75%, and thereby protect the liver against further, large doses of the compound. Various studies have now suggested that, although the initiating event may be formation of the trichloromethyl or similar radical, this is not the major cause of damage. A cascade of events, initiated by radical reactions, is thought to be responsible (figure 7.5).

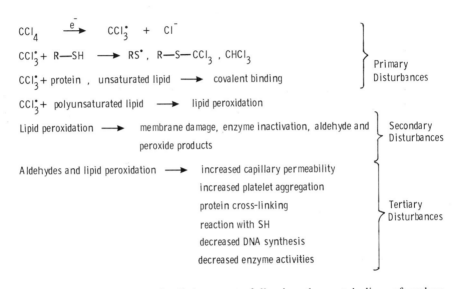

Figure 7.5. The sequence of cellular events following the metabolism of carbon tetrachloride to a reactive free radical.

The first events occurring after a toxic dose of carbon tetrachloride may be observed or detected biochemically around the endoplasmic reticulum. Within one minute of dosing, carbon tetrachloride is covalently bound to microsomal lipid and protein (in the ratio 11 : 3) and conjugated dienes can be detected in lipids within five minutes. These changes in lipids may reflect a transient stage in the alteration of the polyunsaturated fatty acids in the endoplasmic reticulum, but they are not dose-related. Also within the first few minutes after dosing there is evidence that lipid peroxidation occurs. Within 30 minutes to one hour after dosing, protein synthesis is depressed, reflecting changes in the ribosomes and rough endoplasmic reticulum. Also cytochrome P-450 content and activity are decreased, the activity of glucose-6-phosphatase, an enzyme associated with the endoplasmic reticulum, is lowered, as is NADPH content.

Morphologically, changes which can be observed within this time period are confined to the loss of ribosomes from the endoplasmic reticulum, but no other changes are discernible.

One to three hours after dosing with carbon tetrachloride, triglycerides can be seen to accumulate as fat droplets in the liver cell, and the enzymic activities associated with the endoplasmic reticulum continue to fall. Calcium accumulates and is secreted, but this appears to be a transient change. The rough endoplasmic reticulum becomes vacuolated and continues to shed ribosomes, while the smooth endoplasmic reticulum shows signs of membrane collapse, eventually contracting into clumps. At later time-points lysosomal damage may become apparent, when the centrilobular cells are damaged, and cells may begin to show intracellular structural modifications. Eventually the plasma membrane ruptures, although little, if any, evidence of damage to the plasma membrane is apparent before this. This sequence of changes is well defined and common to a number of different species.

As already mentioned, metabolism of carbon tetrachloride by the microsomal mono-oxygenases is necessary for hepatotoxicity, and the product is almost certainly a radical such as the trichloromethyl radical (figure 7.4). This radical may react particularly with SH groups and methylene bridges on polyunsaturated fatty acids. Because of its short half-life its radius of action is small, and probably confined to the immediate vicinity of the cytochrome P-450. Studies *in vitro* have revealed that production of this radical and its covalent interaction with protein occurs in the absence of oxygen, but destruction of cytochrome P-450 and damage to the microsomes, measured *in vitro* as loss of glucose-6-phosphatase activity, only occurs in the presence of oxygen. It therefore seems that the covalent binding of the trichloromethyl radical to cellular constituents may not necessarily be of major importance to the toxicity.

Consequently, it is now generally accepted that the more important event is the production of lipid radicals which, on reaction with oxygen, form peroxides and eventually short-chain aldehydes and hydroxy alkenals as shown in figure 6.9. These events can be followed by monitoring for conjugated dienes, for malondialdehyde (a terminal product of lipid peroxidation) and for alkanes.

It now seems clear that a number of toxicities may be mediated via lipid peroxidation. Therefore, although the trichloromethyl radical may be important in damaging cytochrome P-450 and its immediate vicinity, the more distant cellular targets are almost certainly damaged by the products of lipid peroxidation in a cascade system. The mechanisms underlying the pathological changes are still speculative, but damage to structural lipids, particularly of the smooth and rough endoplasmic reticulum, by lipid radicals and their peroxides, is thought to play a major role. Inhibition of protein synthesis occurs and may be partially responsible for the fatty liver but probably not the necrosis, although it contributes to the general disabling of the cell. Altered membrane function due to direct attack by radicals or from peroxidation products is therefore probably a major event. The various schemes are shown in figure 7.5.

It is clear that both the covalent binding of carbon tetrachloride metabolites to protein and lipid, and lipid peroxidation, result from the metabolic
production of the trichloromethyl radical. The reactions of the trichloromethyl radical or its peroxy derivative may be responsible for the damage to
cytochrome P-450 and its immediate vicinity. The major cellular damage
is, however, probably the result of the lipid radicals produced by the interaction of the trichloromethyl radical with unsaturated lipids and fatty acids.
The cascade of events set in train by these lipid radicals probably includes
membrane damage which may lead to cellular necrosis.

Paracetamol

Paracetamol (acetaminophen) is a widely used analgesic and antipyretic
drug which has remarkably little toxicity when taken at prescribed therapeutic doses. After overdoses of this drug are taken, however, as is becoming
increasingly common in suicide attempts, it causes a centrilobular hepatic
necrosis and in some cases renal damage. Measurement of the plasma level
of paracetamol after overdoses reveals that the patients' ability to conjugate
paracetamol is impaired and that the half-life is extended several-fold
(table 7.1). The plasma half-life of paracetamol has been used to estimate
the severity of liver damage and therefore the type of treatment required.

The hepatic damage is reproducible, and paracetamol administered by
various routes causes hepatic necrosis in many different species of experimental animal, although there is wide species sensitivity. The hepatotoxicity
of paracetamol was found to be markedly increased by pretreatment of
animals with microsomal enzyme inducers such as phenobarbital and conversely reduced in animals given microsomal enzyme inhibitors. Furthermore,
there was a lack of correlation between tissue levels of paracetamol and the

Table 7.1. Mean plasma concentration and half-life of unchanged paracetamol in patients with and without paracetamol-induced liver damage.

Patients	Plasma paracetamol half-life (h)	Plasma paracetamol concentrations (µg/ml)	
		4 h after ingestion	12 h after ingestion
No liver damage (18)	$2 \cdot 9 \pm 0 \cdot 3$	163 ± 20	$29 \cdot 5 \pm 6$
Liver damage (23)	$7 \cdot 2 \pm 0 \cdot 7$	296 ± 26	124 ± 22

Numbers of patients in parentheses.
Data of Prescott & Wright (1973) *Br. J. Pharmac.*, **39**, 602.

Table 7.2. The effect of various pretreatments on the severity of hepatic necrosis from and covalent binding of paracetamol to mouse tissue protein.

Treatment	Dose of Paracetamol (mg/kg)	Severity of liver necrosis[3]	Covalent binding of ^{3}H-Paracetamol (nmol/mg protein)[4]	
			Liver	Muscle
None	375	1–2+	1·02 ± 0·17	0·02 ± 0·02
[1]Piperonyl butoxide	375	0	0·33 ± 0·05	0·01 ± 0·01
[1]Cobaltous chloride	375	0	0·39 ± 0·11	0·01 ± 0·03
α-[1]Naphthylisothiocyanate	375	0	0·11 ± 0·06	0·01 ± 0·02
[2]Phenobarbital	375	2–4±	1·6 ± 0·1	0·02 ± 0·02

[1] Microsomal enzyme inhibitor; [2]microsomal enzyme inducer.
[3] Data of Mitchell *et al.* (1973) *J. Pharmac. exp. Ther.*, **187**, 185; [4] Data from Jollow *et al.* (1973) *J. Pharmac. exp. Ther.*, **187**, 175, and from Mitchell & Jollow (1975) *Gastroenterology*, **58**, 392.
Severity of necrosis: 1+ <6% necrotic hepatocytes; 2+ >6% <25% necrotic hepatocytes; 3+ >25% <50% necrotic hepatocytes; 4+ >50% necrotic hepatocytes.

necrosis. These findings indicated that a metabolite was responsible for the hepatotoxicity rather than the parent drug (table 7.2).

Further studies revealed that when radiolabelled paracetamol was administered to experimental animals it was covalently bound to liver protein. Autoradiography showed that this binding was mainly confined to the necrotic areas of the liver. This covalent binding of paracetamol to liver protein *in vivo* was inversely related to the level of unchanged drug in the liver and was increased or decreased by prior pretreatment of animals with microsomal enzyme inducers or inhibitors respectively (table 7.2). The extent of covalent binding increased markedly with increasing dosage and the binding was time-dependent in the liver whereas the minimal, background binding to muscle protein was not.

These findings confirmed the involvement of a reactive metabolite of paracetamol rather than the drug itself. However, the metabolic profile of paracetamol is simple and straightforward (figure 7.6), involving glucuronic acid and sulphate conjugation as major pathways, with a small amount (5% dose in man) of a mercapturic acid or *N*-acetylcysteine conjugate being excreted. None of these metabolites are chemically reactive or likely to react with liver protein.

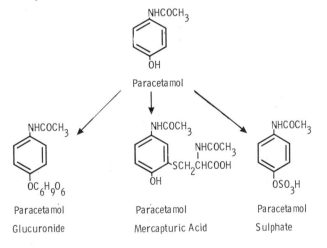

Figure 7.6. The major metabolites of paracetamol.

However, measurement of the mercapturic acid excreted in the urine after different doses of paracetamol indicated that the excretion of the conjugate was reduced after toxic doses of paracetamol and at the same time hepatic glutathione was depleted to about 20% or less of the normal level (figure 7.7). Thus there was an apparent relationship between the metabolism, covalent binding and liver glutathione level. These observations lead to the proposed scheme shown in figure 7.8.

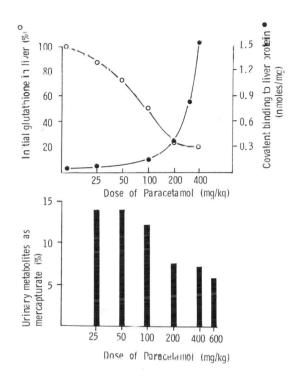

Figure 7.7. Relationship between hepatic glutathione, covalent binding of radio-labelled Paracetamol to hepatic protein and urinary excretion of Paracetamol mercapturic acid after different doses of paracetamol. Adapted from Mitchell *et al.* (1975). In *Handbook of Experimental Pharmacology*, Vol. 28, Part 3, *Concepts in Biochemical Pharmacology*, edited by J. R. Gillette and J. R. Mitchell (Berlin: Springer Verlag).

The reactive intermediate is generally believed to be the *N*-acetylimido-quinone, although the preceding step from which it arises is still controversial. It almost certainly involves oxidation of the nitrogen. Studies *in vitro* established that the production of the reactive intermediate of paracetamol involved the cytochrome P-450 dependent mono-oxygenases. Using covalent binding as a measure of production of the reactive metabolite, it was shown that the activation required NADPH and oxygen and was inhibited by carbon monoxide. Using ^{18}O in similar studies, it was shown that no ^{18}O was incorporated, indicating that the reactive intermediate was not an epoxide.

The proposed mechanism of paracetamol hepatotoxicity therefore involved metabolic activation to a reactive intermediate which was detoxified by conjugation with glutathione, both enzymically and chemically. This normally adequate detoxication pathway is overloaded after large toxic doses, so the hepatic level of glutathione is reduced more rapidly than it can be replenished.

The result is that the reactive metabolite reacts with various hepatic macro-molecules and this in some as yet unknown way gives rise to hepatic necrosis. Thus there is a marked toxic dose threshold which occurs when glutathione levels are at a minimum.

Although this elegant scheme explains the experimental observations, it is not yet clear how the covalent binding of the reactive intermediate precipi-tates hepatic necrosis. More recent data suggests that covalent binding may be only one of a series of events involved in the pathogenesis of the lesion. Protection of animals and man from paracetamol hepatotoxicity may be afforded by sulphydryl agents such as cysteamine and *N*-acetylcysteine. However, this is effective at times after dosing when animal data suggests that covalent binding to hepatic protein has already reached its maximum.

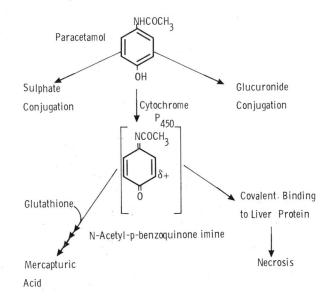

Figure 7.8. Proposed metabolic activation of paracetamol to a toxic, reactive intermediate which may be detoxified by conjugation with glutathione or which may react with tissue proteins when glutathione is depleted.

There are marked species differences in paracetamol hepatotoxicity due to variation in microsomal enzyme activity. The hamster is several times more sensitive to paracetamol hepatotoxicity than the rat. Pretreatment of hamsters with phenobarbital, however, decreases the hepatotoxicity, unlike the case in rats and mice where the toxicity is increased. This is thought to be due to the induction of glucuronidation, a detoxication pathway (figure 7.8), by phenobarbital to a greater extent than induction of the microsomal enzymes responsible for the toxic pathway. However, 3-methylcholanthrene

(3MC) pretreatment increases hepatotoxicity, suggesting that a 3MC-inducible form of cytochrome P-450 may be involved in the metabolic activation of paracetamol in the hamster.

As well as induction of the microsomal enzymes, there are other factors which increase toxicity. Depletion of hepatic glutathione with compounds such as diethyl maleate (figure 4.55) lowers the toxic dose threshold by removing hepatic protection in the form of detoxication capacity. Inhibition of the pathways of glucuronidation and sulphation with compounds such as salicylamide increase toxicity by diverting more of the drug down the toxic pathway (figure 7.8).

It now seems possible that depletion of glutathione, not in itself a sufficient insult, coupled with covalent binding and possible damage to various membrane proteins may lead to loss of NADP(H) and NAD(H) and an inability of the afflicted cell to function. However, it is clear that much research remains to be done on this fascinating interface between biochemical toxicology and pathology.

The elucidation of the mechanism underlying paracetamol toxicity is particularly significant in that it has led to a successful method of treatment for overdose cases. Various sulphydryl donors have been tried as possible antidotes and the use of intravenous *N*-acetylcysteine is now well established as a successful mode of treatment for overdosage in man, provided it is used within ten hours of overdosing.

Bromobenzene

Bromobenzene is a toxic industrial solvent, doses of which cause centrilobular hepatic necrosis in experimental animals, and in some cases bronchiolar necrosis may also be produced. The metabolism of bromobenzene involves epoxidation at the 3,4 position (figure 7.9) and the product of this, the 3,4-epoxide, is detoxified with glutathione, to be excreted as a mercapturic acid. Also the epoxide rearranges to 4-bromophenol and is hydrated by epoxide hydratase to yield the dihydrodiol (figure 7.9). It was found that radiolabelled bromobenzene was covalently bound to liver protein after toxic doses of the radiolabelled compound were given to experimental animals. Furthermore it was observed that this covalent binding to liver protein and the hepatic necrosis were increased by pretreatment of animals with phenobarbital, the microsomal enzyme inducer, but decreased by inhibitors of these enzymes.

As the major route of metabolism was believed to be microsomal metabolism to bromobenzene epoxide, it was reasoned that the pretreatment with phenobarbital should simply increase the rate of formation of the epoxide, not the total amount. As this induction of the microsomal enzymes increased the hepatotoxicity of bromobenzene, other time-dependent factors were

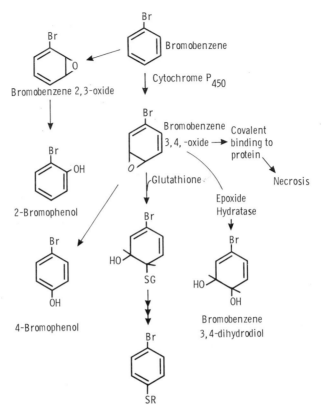

Figure 7.9. Metabolism of bromobenzene. The bromobenzene 2,3-oxide and 3,4-oxide may undergo chemical rearrangement to the 2- and 4-bromophenol respectively. Bromobenzene 3,4-oxide may also be conjugated with glutathione and in its absence react with tissue proteins. An alternative, detoxication pathway is hydration to the 3,4-dihydrodiol via epoxide hydratase.

obviously involved. This reasoning led to the discovery that the level of hepatic glutathione was a major factor, being markedly depleted by toxic doses of bromobenzene (figure 7.10). Glutathione conjugation is a detoxication reaction, removing the reactive epoxide intermediate which would otherwise arylate tissue macromolecules. Consequently, a deficiency of this co-substrate leaves the liver unprotected, and exposure to bromobenzene results in hepatotoxicity. Hydration of the epoxide to the dihydrodiol is also a detoxication pathway, as is chemical rearrangement to 4-bromophenol (figure 7.9).

A particularly interesting finding to emerge from this work was the effect of pretreatment of animals with 3-methylcholanthrene. Unexpectedly this

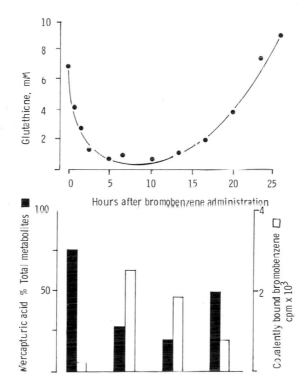

Figure 7.10. Relationship between hepatic glutathione, covalent binding of radio-labelled bromobenzene to hepatic protein and urinary excretion of bromophenyl mercapturic acid in rats. Animals were given bromobenzene (10 mmol/kg, i.p.) and then radiolabelled bromobenzene at various times thereafter. Adapted from Gillette (1973) *5th Int. Congr. Pharmacology*, Vol. 2 (Basel: Karger).

was found to reduce the hepatotoxicity of bromobenzene. This effect seems to be due to two changes caused by 3-methylcholanthrene treatment (table 7.3):

(*a*) Increased activity of the epoxide hydratase enzyme which detoxifies bromobenzene by hydration to the diol;

(*b*) Increased metabolism of bromobenzene to the 2,3-epoxide intermediate, which more readily undergoes rearrangement to bromophenol than the 3,4-epoxide (figure 7.9).

The result of these two changes is therefore less tissue arylation by the 3,4-epoxide and hence less hepatic necrosis.

The interrelationship between glutathione levels and metabolic pathways has been elegantly shown both *in vivo* and *in vitro*. In vivo the dependence of urinary mercapturic acid excretion, hepatic glutathione concentration and covalent binding and their relationship to hepatic necrosis is clear

Table 7.3. Effect of 3-methylcholanthrene (3-MC) pretreatment on the urinary metabolites of bromobenzene.

Metabolites	% Total urinary metabolites	
	Untreated	3-MC treated
4-Bromophenylmercapturic acid	72	31
4-Bromophenol	14	20
4-Bromocatechol	6	10
4-Bromophenyldihydrodiol	3	17
2-Bromophenol	4	21

Data from Zampaglione *et al.* (1973) *J. Pharmac. exp. Ther.*, **187**, 218.
Dose of bromobenzene 10 mmol/kg to rats.

(figure 7.10). Studies *in vitro* using the S-9 fraction from rat liver homogenates similarly showed the importance of the glutathione concentration; all the hydroxylated metabolites and covalently bound bromobenzene were reduced by increasing levels of glutathione, but the total level of metabolism remained constant.

Although autoradiography indicates that the majority of the covalent binding in the liver is to necrotic hepatocytes in the centrilobular region, the nature of the binding is not yet clear. Studies in isolated hepatocytes have indicated that although binding to the microsomal fraction is greatest, the reactive metabolite does migrate into the cytosol and bind at other sites. Bromobenzene is cytotoxic in isolated hepatocytes but the cells are protected by glutathione, depletion of which precedes other signs of toxicity. As well as binding to protein, arylation of other low molecular weight nucleophiles such as pyridine nucleotides and CoA also occurs. Glutathione depletion is accounted for by the formation of conjugates; lipid peroxidation and subsequent oxidation of glutathione do not seem to be involved in this depletion. There are also indications that some of the phenolic metabolites may be hepatotoxic after further metabolic activation.

In conclusion, bromobenzene hepatotoxicity is due to metabolic activation to a reactive epoxide which arylates tissue macromolecules. As with some of the other examples in this section, however, the sequence of events which follows this covalent interaction with proteins and other macromolecules and the exact relationship with the hepatic necrosis which ensues is still unclear.

Isoniazid and iproniazid

Isoniazid and iproniazid are chemically similar drugs having different pharmacological effects; they may both cause liver damage after therapeutic doses are given. Isoniazid is still widely used for the treatment of tuberculosis, but iproniazid is now rarely used as an antidepressant.

Isoniazid-related mild hepatic dysfunction is now well recognized as occurring in 10–20% of recipients of the drug. Up to 1% of these cases progress to severe hepatic damage. Initial evidence that the incidence of hepatic damage was greater in the rapid acetylator phenotype (see page 102), prompted a study of the relationship between metabolism and toxicity.

The major routes of metabolism for isoniazid are acetylation to give acetylisoniazid, followed by hydrolysis to yield isonicotinic acid and acetylhydrazine (figure 7.11). The acetylation of isoniazid has a genetic component, (see page 102), human populations being divisible into rapid and slow acetylator phenotypes depending upon the amount of acetylisoniazid

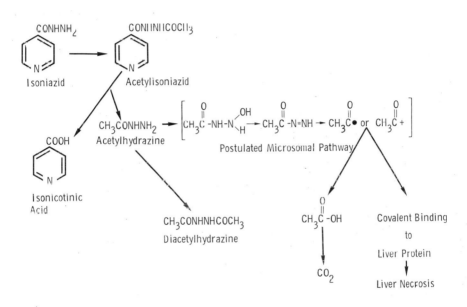

Figure 7.11. Metabolism of isoniazid. The acetylhydrazine released by the hydrolysis of acetylisoniazid is further metabolized to a reactive intermediate thought to be responsible for the hepatotoxicity.

excreted. Animal studies revealed that both acetylisoniazid and acetylhydrazine were hepatotoxic, causing centrilobular necrosis in phenobarbital-pretreated animals. Conversely, pretreatment of animals with microsomal enzyme inhibitors reduced necrosis. Inhibition of the hydrolysis of acetylisoniazid (figure 7.11) with bis-p-nitrophenylphosphate (figure 5.21), an acyl amidase inhibitor, reduced its hepatotoxicity, but not that of acetylhydrazine. Further studies revealed that metabolism of acetylhydrazine by the microsomal mono-oxygenases was responsible for the hepatotoxicity, resulting in the covalent binding of the acetyl group to liver protein. This data indicated that acetylhydrazine was the toxic metabolite produced from acetylisoniazid,

Table 7.4. Effect of various pretreatments on the hepatotoxicity, covalent binding and metabolism to CO_2 of acetylisoniazid and acetylhydrazine.

Pretreatment	Acetylisoniazid (200 mg/kg)			Acetylhydrazine (20 mg/kg)		
	[4]Necrosis	[5]Covalent binding (nmol/mg protein)	[5] [14]CO_2 (% Dose)	[4]Necrosis (30 mg/kg)	[5]Covalent binding (nmol/mg protein)	[5] [14]CO_2 (% Dose)
None	0+	0·20	10	0+	0·15	29
[1]Phenobarbital	++	0·31	12	+++	0·19	35
Phenobarbital+ [2]Cobalt chloride	0	0·15	4	0	0·09	22
Phenobarbital+ [3]bis-p-nitrophenyl phosphate	0	0·11	4	+++	0·23	37

[1] Microsomal enzyme inducer; [2] microsomal enzyme inhibitor; [3] acylamidase inhibitor.
[4] Data from Mitchell *et al.* (1976) *Ann. Intern. Med.*, **84**, 181.
[5] Data from Timbrell *et al.* (1980) *J. Pharmac. exp. Ther.*, **213**, 364.
Severity of necrosis: 1+ <6% necrotic hepatocytes; 2+ >6% <25% necrotic hepatocytes; 3+ >25% <50% necrotic hepatocytes; 4+ >50% necrotic hepatocytes.

and therefore isoniazid. Acetylhydrazine required metabolic activation via the microsomal enzymes to a reactive acylating intermediate which would react with protein (table 7.4).

The proposed activation of acetylhydrazine involves N-hydroxylation, followed by loss of water to yield acetyldiazine, an intermediate which would fragment to yield acetyl radical or acetyl carbonium ion (figure 7.11). Glutathione was not depleted by hepatotoxic doses of acetylhydrazine, indicating that unlike bromobenzene or paracetamol toxicity, it does not have a direct protective role.

The role of acetylhydrazine in isoniazid hepatotoxicity is complex, as the production of the toxic intermediate involves several steps. Further study has indicated that acetylhydrazine is detoxified by further acetylation to diacetylhydrazine (figure 7.11) and that isoniazid may interact with acetylhydrazine metabolism. It is therefore clear that the relative rates of production, detoxication and activation of acetylhydrazine are very important determinants of the hepatotoxicity of isoniazid.

The acetylation of isoniazid and acetylhydrazine are both subject to genetic variability, so the production and detoxication pathways are both influenced by the acetylator phenotype. The hepatotoxicity of isoniazid is therefore dependent on a complex interrelationship between genetic factors and individual variation in the pharmacokinetics of isoniazid.

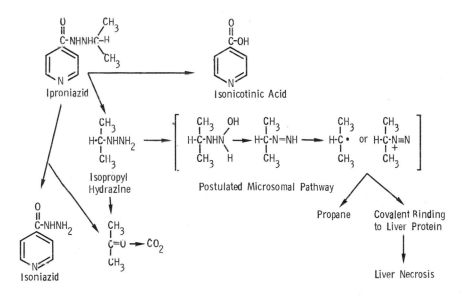

Figure 7.12. Metabolism of iproniazid. The isopropylhydrazine moiety released by hydrolysis is further metabolized to a reactive intermediate thought to be responsible for the hepatotoxicity.

Iproniazid hepatotoxicity has a similar basis to that of isoniazid toxicity. Hydrolysis of iproniazid yields isopropylhydrazine (figure 7.12) which is extremely hepatotoxic in experimental animals. Isopropylhydrazine is metabolically activated by the microsomal enzymes to a reactive alkylating species which covalently binds to liver protein. One of the products of this metabolic route has been shown to be propane gas, the presence of which indicates that the isopropyl radical may be the reactive intermediate. This was further suggested by double labelling experiments, which showed that the whole isopropyl moiety is bound to protein without loss of hydrogen atoms (figure 7.12). Sulphydryl compounds reduce the covalent binding to protein *in vitro*, and *S*-isopropyl conjugates have been isolated from preparations *in vitro*, which confirms the role of the isopropyl group as an alkylating species. However, sulphydryl compounds are not depleted *in vivo* by hepatotoxic doses of isopropylhydrazine.

Thus the hepatotoxicity of iproniazid and isoniazid almost certainly involves the alkylation of tissue proteins and other macromolecules in the liver. How these covalent interactions lead to the observed hepatocellular necrosis is at present not understood.

Tissue lesions: lung damage

4-Ipomeanol

4-Ipomeanol (figure 7.13) is a pulmonary toxin produced by the mould *Fusarium solani*, which grows on sweet potatoes. The pure compound produces lung damage in a number of species when given intraperitoneally. This lung damage is manifested as oedema, congestion and haemorrhage. These are probably secondary or tertiary pathological changes resulting from the primary lesion, which is necrosis of the non-ciliated bronchiolar cells, also known as the Clara cells. Toxicologically, 4-ipomeanol is of particular interest as it is a specific lung toxin which selectively damages one cell type, the Clara cell.

The elucidation of the mechanism has revealed that this specificity is due to a requirement for metabolic activation for which the Clara cell is particularly suited. Using radiolabelled 4-ipomeanol it was found that the compound

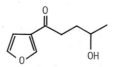

Figure 7.13. Structure of 4-ipomeanol.

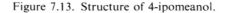

was localized particularly in the lungs (when expressed as nmol/g wet weight of tissue), and was covalently bound to lung protein. This binding was five times that seen in the liver. Furthermore, autoradiography revealed that the radiolabelled 4-ipomeanol was bound to the Clara cells, which were necrotic, whereas ciliated and other cells lining the airways did not show necrosis or covalently bound radioactivity.

Studies *in vitro* showed that 4-ipomeanol was metabolically activated by the microsomal mono-oxygenases to an alkylating species which would covalently interact with protein. Although the level of cytochrome P-450 in the lung is lower than that in the liver, the V_{max} for the covalent binding to lung microsomal protein was higher than that for liver. Glutathione inhibited the binding to protein *in vitro*.

Studies *in vivo* indicated that the cause of death was probably pulmonary oedema, as the time-course for lethality and oedemagenesis were similar (figure 7.14). Also, the pulmonary oedema and lethality showed a very similar dose–response and the covalent binding to pulmonary protein was similarly dose-dependent (figure 7.15).

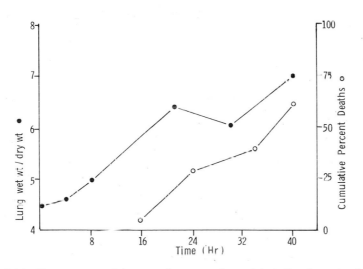

Figure 7.14. Time-course of lung oedemagenesis and lethality in animals given 4-ipomeanol. Adapted from Boyd *et al.* (1978) *J. Pharmac. exp. Ther.*, **207**, 687.

Inhibitors of the microsomal enzymes decreased the covalent binding and the Clara cell necrosis and increased the LD_{50} even though the blood and pulmonary levels of ipomeanol were increased. The microsomal enzyme inducer phenobarbital decreased binding to both liver and lung protein and correspondingly increased the LD_{50}. In contrast, 3-methylcholanthrene induction increased binding in the liver and potentiated liver necrosis, but again decreased lung binding and lung damage. The LD_{50} was again increased.

Diethyl maleate treatment, which depletes glutathione, markedly increased covalent binding to protein and decreased the LD_{50}. Analogues of 4-ipomeanol in which the furan ring was replaced by a methyl or phenyl group were very much less toxic and did not covalently bind to lung or liver protein to any great extent.

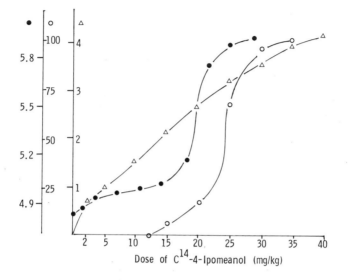

Figure 7.15. Dose–response curves for lethality (%, ○), oedemagenesis (wet weight : dry weight ratios, ●) and pulmonary covalent binding (nmol/mg protein, △) of radiolabelled 4-ipomeanol given i.p. to the rat. Adapted from Boyd *et al.* (1978) *J. Pharmac. exp. Ther.*, **207**, 687.

There is good correlation between the toxicity as measured by lethality or LD_{50}, oedemagenesis and covalent binding of radiolabelled ipomeanol to protein (figure 7.15). The reason for the pulmonary selectivity is not yet clear, but liver necrosis may occur if hepatic metabolic activation is increased by 3-methylcholanthrene treatment. The particular susceptibility of the Clara cell in the lung could reflect a deficiency in protective mechanisms as well as the level of microsomal enzyme activity. It seems likely that the metabolic activation takes place *in situ* rather than the reactive metabolite being transported from the liver.

In conclusion, the pulmonary toxicity of 4-ipomeanol seems to be due to metabolic activation of the furan ring, probably by epoxidation, catalysed by the cytochrome P-450 mono-oxygenases found in the Clara cell. The reactive intermediate binds to protein and possibly other macromolecules, initiating cellular necrosis followed by oedema.

Neurotoxicity

Isoniazid

As well as being implicated as a hepatotoxin, the antituberculous drug isoniazid may also cause peripheral neuropathy with chronic use. In practice this can be avoided by the concomitant administration of vitamin B_6 (pyridoxine).

In experimental animals, however, chronic dosing with isoniazid causes degeneration of the peripheral nerves. The biochemical basis for this involves interference with vitamin B_6 metabolism. Isoniazid reacts with pyridoxal phosphate to form a hydrazone (figure 7.16) which is a very potent inhibitor of pyridoxal phosphate kinase. The hydrazone has a much greater affinity for the enzyme (100 1000 ×) than the normal substrate, pyridoxal. The result of this is a depletion of tissue pyridoxal phosphate. This cofactor is of importance particularly in nervous tissue for reactions involving decarboxylation and transamination. The decarboxylation reactions are principally affected however, with the result that transamination reactions assume a greater importance.

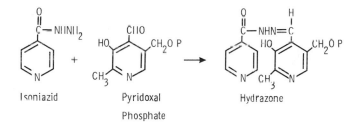

Figure 7.16. Reaction of isoniazid with pyridoxal phosphate to form a hydrazone.

In man peripheral neuropathy due to isoniazid is influenced by the acetylator phenotype (see page 102), being predominantly found in slow acetylators. This is probably due to the higher plasma level of isoniazid in this phenotype. In this case, therefore, acetylation is a detoxication reaction, removing the isoniazid and rendering it unreactive towards pyridoxal phosphate, in contrast to the situation with the hepatotoxicity

6-Hydroxydopamine

6-Hydroxydopamine is a selectively neurotoxic compound which damages the sympathetic nerve endings. It can be seen from figure 7.17 that 6-hydroxydopamine is structurally very similar to dopamine and noradrenaline.

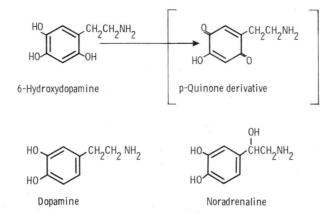

Figure 7.17. Structures of dopamine and noradrenaline, the analogue 6-hydroxy-dopamine and a possible oxidation product.

and because of this it is actively taken up into the synaptic system along with other catecholamines. Once localized in the synapse the 6-hydroxydopamine destroys the nerve terminal. A single small dose of 6-hydroxydopamine destroys all the nerve terminals and possibly the nerve cells as well.

The mechanism of the destruction of the nerve terminals is thought to involve oxidation of 6-hydroxydopamine to a *p*-quinone, the production of a free radical or of superoxide anion. It seems that a reactive intermediate is produced which reacts covalently with the nerve terminal and permanently inactivates it.

Factors which influence the disposition of catecholamines will affect the toxicity. For instance, compounds which inhibit the uptake of noradrenaline reduce the destruction of adrenergic nerve terminals but not of dopaminergic ones. Interference with the oxidative metabolism of catecholamines also influences the toxicity of 6-hydroxydopamine.

This example of selective neurotoxicity particularly illustrates the potential importance of the distribution of a foreign compound in the type and localization of the toxic effect it causes.

Exaggerated and unwanted pharmacological effects

The exaggerated or unwanted pharmacological responses are the most common toxic effects of drugs observed clinically, as opposed to direct toxic effects on tissues. However, this type of response may also be observed with other compounds such as the toxic cholinesterase inhibitors used as pesticides and nerve gases.

Cholinesterase inhibitors

There are many different cholinesterase inhibitors which find use particularly as insecticides but also as nerve gases for chemical warfare. The toxic effects are due to the inhibition of acetylcholinesterase, an enzyme found in the plasma and other tissues, which hydrolyses acetylcholine to choline and acetate (figure 7.18). This hydrolysis effectively terminates the action of acetylcholine, which is a chemical transmitter active at the synaptic nerve

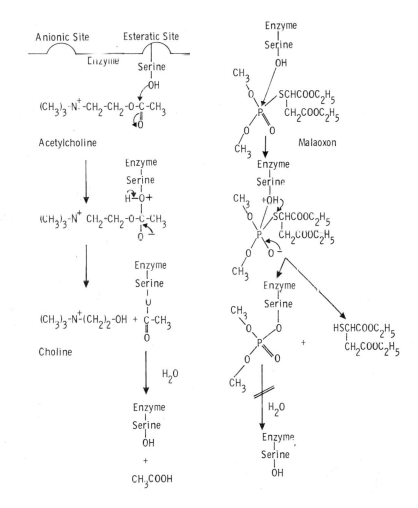

Figure 7.18. Mechanism of hydrolysis of acetylcholine by acetylcholinesterase and blockade of the enzyme by malaoxon. With malaoxon as substrate, the final step, regeneration of the enzyme by hydrolysis, is blocked ($\neq$) leading to inactivated enzyme.

endings in the nervous system, glands and smooth muscle. The symptoms of toxicity are the result of excessive cholinergic stimulation due to accumulation of acetylcholine. When the activity of acetylcholinesterase is reduced to 50% toxic effects ensue and at 10–20% of normal activity (80–90% inhibition) death follows. The cause of death is usually respiratory failure, due partly to neuromuscular paralysis and partly to central depression.

Organophosphorus cholinesterase inhibitors may also damage the peripheral nerves, causing degeneration, muscular weakness and sensory disturbances. An example of this is tri-orthocresyl phosphate (TOCP) (figure 2.9) which, although not a potent cholinesterase inhibitor, produces delayed neurotoxic effects. The relationship between this toxic effect and the cholinesterase activity is not clear, but may involve a different mechanism. The inhibition of acetylcholinesterase, which relies on the inhibitor being a pseudosubstrate for the enzyme, is reversible but the rate of regeneration may be very slow, with a half-life of 10–30 days.

Many of the cholinesterase inhibitors are rapidly metabolized or excreted *in vivo* and do not generally accumulate. However, a cumulative toxic effect may occur by virtue of the long half-life of regeneration of the enzyme, so chronic dosing may eventually cause sufficient cumulative inhibition to produce toxicity. The majority of cholinesterase inhibitors are esters, phosphate esters being the most common, but some carbamates are also potent inhibitors. In some cases inhibitors used as insecticides have been devised which have low mammalian toxicity compared with the toxicity in the target organism. This can be done by exploiting differences in metabolism. For example, malathion is relatively non-toxic to mammals but an effective insecticide. In mammals the major route of metabolism is hydrolysis and

Acetylcholinesterase Catalysis

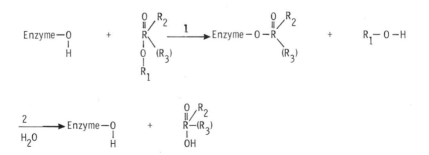

Figure 7.19. General scheme for acetylcholinesterase action. R may $= C$ or P. If $R = P$, then (R_3) is present. The group OR_1 may be replaced by SR_1, giving R_1SH on hydrolysis (reaction 1). If $R = P$, reaction 2 is very slow, giving inactivated enzyme. The rate of hydrolysis or reactivation depends on the nature of R_2 and R_3.

excretion of the product as conjugates. In insects, however, oxidative desulphuration occurs, producing malaoxon which is a potent cholinesterase inhibitor (figures 5.7 and 7.18).

Mechanism of inhibition

Inhibition of cholinesterases depends upon blockade of the active site of the enzyme, specifically the site which binds the ester portion of the acetylcholine (figure 7.18). The inhibitor or pseudosubstrate becomes bound at the active site, and undergoes cleavage to release the corresponding alcohol or thiol, leaving a phosphorylated or carbamylated enzyme (figure 7.19). The hydrolysis of this enzyme intermediate is slow, however, unlike that of the normal intermediate, which is the acetylated enzyme. This is illustrated by comparing the normal substrate acetylcholine with the inhibitor malaoxon (figure 7.18). The general reaction is therefore:

Cholinesterase + Substrate→Acetylated enzyme + Product
(Inhibitor)   (Phosphorylated or
          carbamylated enzyme)

Fast hydrolysis→Regenerated enzyme
(Slow)   (Regenerated enzyme)

The esteratic site contains a serine hydroxyl group which interacts with the carbonyl carbon atom of acetylcholine or the phosphorus atom of organophosphate inhibitors (figure 7.19). This allows cleavage of the ester bond, followed by spontaneous hydrolysis of the acetylated enzyme, to regenerate the serine hydroxyl and thus the active form of the enzyme. The phosphorylated or carbamylated enzyme is only slowly hydrolysed and the esteratic site is therefore effectively blocked (figures 7.18 and 7.19).

The toxicity will therefore ultimately depend on the affinity of the enzyme for the inhibitor and the rate of hydrolysis of the phosphorylated or carbamylated intermediate. The production of the inhibitor from an inactive precursor, as is the case with malathion, will also be a determining factor. It is clear from figure 5.7 that malathion could undergo numerous routes of metabolism, and the relative importance of these compared with desulphuration are important determinants of the ultimate toxicity.

Digitalis glycosides

Some of the toxic effects of the digitalis glycosides have been known since digitalis was first described by William Withering in 1785. Overdoses cause vomiting, diarrhoea, visual disturbances, hypotension, slow pulse and ventricular tachycardia, eventually leading to ventricular fibrillation, delirium and convulsions. Toxic effects such as vomiting are not infrequent in the clinical use of the drug, as it has a narrow margin of safety, or a low therapeutic ratio. The dose is therefore critical for any given patient, and monitoring the plasma level of the drug may be necessary to avoid toxicity.

There is wide individual variation in the response to digitalis, which has a long half-life and which therefore may accumulate when certain dose regimens are used. This accumulation, the low therapeutic index (see page 16) and the individual variation in response are responsible for the toxicity encountered in the normal clinical use of the drug. It can be seen from figure 7.20 that digitoxin (one of the digitalis glycosides) will be toxic, causing vomiting, in 3 out of 100 patients at the ED_{50} dose. The dose therefore has to be individualized to try to avoid this.

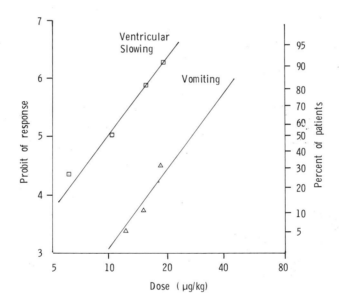

Figure 7.20. Comparison of the pharmacological and toxic effects of digitoxin in man. The pharmacological effect was a 40–50% decrease in heart rate; the toxic effect, nausea and vomiting, occurred after a single oral dose. Adapted from Marsh (1951) *Outline of Fundamental Pharmacology* (Springfield, Ill.: Charles C. Thomas).

The mechanism of action of digitalis glycosides and the mechanisms underlying the toxicity are poorly understood. It seems, however, that toxic doses of digoxin, for instance, cause disturbances in the movement of cations in cardiac tissue, possibly by interacting with an ATPase. Toxic doses cause an efflux of potassium ions from the heart tissue, and therefore an infusion of K^+ may be used as an antidote to the toxicity. The manifestations of toxicity are gastrointestinal disturbances giving rise to nausea, vomiting and diarrhoea, central effects, neurologic and ophthalmologic disorders and cardiac arrhythmias. The pattern of toxic effects is variable but may occur after only a small change in the dose or plasma level.

Diphenylhydantoin

As with the digitalis glycosides, the toxic effects of the anticonvulsant drug diphenylhydantoin result from elevated plasma levels of the drug. This can simply be due to inappropriate dosage, but other factors may also be involved in the development of toxicity.

The toxic effects observed are nystagmus, ataxia, drowsiness and sometimes more serious effects on the CNS. These toxic effects are clearly dose-related and correlate well with the plasma levels of the unchanged drug. High plasma levels may be the result of defective metabolism as well as of excessive dosage (see page 104). Diphenylhydantoin is metabolized by hydroxylation of the aromatic ring (figure 7.21) and this is the major route of metabolism. However, a genetic trait has been described in man in which there appears to be a deficiency in this metabolic route. The consequences of this are decreased metabolism and the appearance of toxicity after therapeutic doses, due to the elevated plasma levels of the unchanged drug.

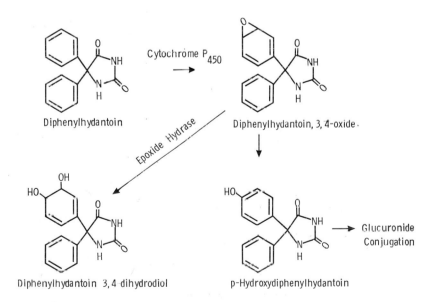

Figure 7.21. Metabolism of diphenylhydantoin.

Another cause of toxicity is the co-administration of other drugs such as isoniazid. This drug, even after normal doses are given, inhibits the hydroxylation of diphenylhydantoin and thereby increases the plasma level of the unchanged drug, leading to toxicity in the same way as described above. The slow acetylator phenotype may be more susceptible to this drug interaction, as the plasma level of isoniazid is higher in this phenotype and therefore the extent of inhibition of hydroxylation is greater.

Succinylcholine

Succinylcholine is a neuromuscular blocking agent which is used clinically to cause muscle relaxation. Its duration of action is short, this being due to rapid metabolism by pseudocholinesterases located in the plasma and liver (figure 7.22). However, in some patients the effect is excessive, with prolonged muscle relaxation and apnea lasting as long as two hours compared to the normal duration of a few minutes.

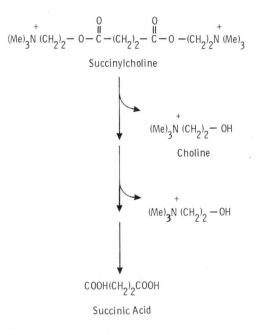

Figure 7.22. Metabolism of succinylcholine by pseudocholinesterases.

This occasional toxicity is due to a deficiency in the hydrolysis of succinylcholine; therefore the parent drug circulates unchanged for longer periods of time and consequently the pharmacological effect is prolonged. This lack of hydrolysis is due to the presence of an atypical pseudocholinesterase.

This aberrant enzyme hydrolyses various substrates, including succinyl-choline, at greatly reduced rates and its affinity for both substrates and inhibitors is markedly different from that of the normal enzyme.

This genetically determined characteristic is found in about 2% of the population, and is absent from certain ethnic groups. The frequencies are consistent with the presence of two allelic autosomal autonomous genes. Consequently, there are both homozygotes and heterozygotes for the abnormal gene, and homozygotes for the normal gene. The heterozygotes for the abnormal gene produce a mixture of normal and abnormal enzyme, and therefore treatment with succinylcholine gives an intermediate response.

Lethal synthesis and incorporation

Fluoroacetate

Monofluoroacetic acid (fluoracetate, figure 7.23) is a compound found naturally in certain South African plants, and which causes severe toxicity in animals eating such plants. The compound has also been used as a rodenticide. The toxicity of fluoroacetate was one of the first to be studied at a basic biochemical level, and Peters coined the term lethal synthesis to describe this biochemical lesion.

Fluoroacetate does not cause direct tissue damage and is not intrinsically toxic but requires metabolism to fluoroacetyl CoA (figure 7.23). Other fluorinated compounds which are metabolized to fluoroacetyl CoA therefore produce the same toxic effects. For instance, compounds such as fluoro-ethanol and fluorofatty acids with even numbers of carbon atoms may undergo β-oxidation to yield fluoroacetyl CoA.

Fluoroacetyl CoA is incorporated into the tricarboxylic acid cycle (TCA cycle) in an analogous manner to acetyl CoA, combining with oxaloacetate to give fluorocitrate (figure 7.23). However, fluorocitrate inhibits the next enzyme of the TCA cycle, aconitase, and there is a buildup of both fluoro-citrate and citrate. The TCA cycle is blocked and the mitochondrial energy supply is disrupted. The inhibition arises from the fact that the aconitase is able to bind fluorocitrate but cannot carry out the dehydration to *cis*-aconitate (figure 7.23). Fluorocitrate is therefore a pseudosubstrate.

The toxicity is manifested as a malfunction of the CNS and heart, giving rise to nausea, apprehension, convulsions and defects of cardiac rhythm, leading to ventricular fibrillation. Fluoroacetate and fluorocitrate do not appear to inhibit other enzymes involved in intermediary metabolism, and the di- and tri-fluoroacetic acids are not similarly incorporated and therefore do not produce the same toxic effects.

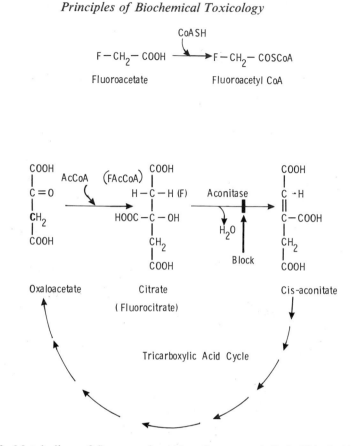

Figure 7.23. Metabolism of fluoroacetic acid to fluoroacetyl CoA (FAcCoA) and mechanism underlying blockade of the tricarboxylic acid cycle. Fluorocitrate cannot be dehydrated to *cis*-aconitate by aconitase and therefore blocks the cycle at this point.

Galactosamine

D-galactosamine is an amino sugar (figure 7.24) normally found *in vivo* only in acetylated form in certain structural polysaccharides. Administration of single doses of this compound to certain species results in a dose-dependent hepatic damage resembling viral hepatitis, with focal necrosis and periportal inflammation. A number of biochemical events have been found to occur. RNA and protein synthesis are inhibited, membrane damage can be observed two hours after dosing and an associated influx of calcium occurs. Also, levels of uridine triphosphate (UTP) and uridine diphosphate glucose (UDP-glucose) fall dramatically within the first hour after the administration of galactosamine. There is also a concomitant rise in UDP-hexosamines and UDP-*N*-acetylhexosamines (figure 7.25).

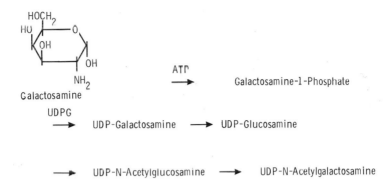

Figure 7.24. Metabolism of galactosamine.

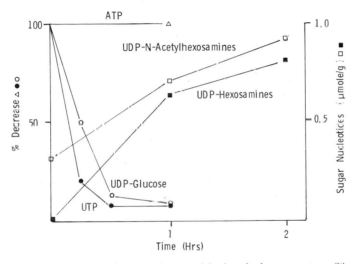

Figure 7.25. The effect of galactosamine on biochemical parameters. The graph shows the effect on ATP ($\triangle$), UTP ($\bullet$), UDP-glucose ($\circ$), UDP-N-acetylhexosamines ($\square$) and UDP-hexosamines ($\blacksquare$). Adapted from Decker & Kepler (1974) *Rev. Physiol. Biochem. Pharmac.*, **71**, 78.

The rapid and extensive depletion of UTP is thought to be the basic cause of the toxicity. Galactosamine combines with UDP to form UDP-galactosamine (figure 7.24), which sequesters UDP, and therefore does not allow cycling of uridine nucleotides. Consequently, synthesis of RNA and hence protein are depressed and sugar and mucopolysaccharide metabolism are disrupted. The latter effects may possibly explain the membrane damage which occurs. The toxic effects of galactosamine can be alleviated by the administration of UTP or its precursors.

Abnormal incorporation of hexosamines into membrane glycoproteins or glycolipids and a concomitant decrease in glucose and galactose incorporation may contribute to membrane damage, and the abnormal entry of calcium in the cell may play a role in the pathogenesis of the lesion. It is of interest, however, that although the mechanism may be compared with that of ethionine hepatotoxicity as described below, the eventual lesions are different. With ethionine the lesion is fatty liver in contrast to the hepatic necrosis caused by galactosamine, although fatty liver may also occur with galactosamine.

Ethionine

Ethionine is a hepatotoxic analogue of the amino acid methionine (figure 7.26). Ethionine is an antimetabolite which has similar chemical and physical properties to the naturally occurring amino acid. After acute doses ethionine causes fatty liver but prolonged administration results in liver cirrhosis and hepatic carcinoma. Some of the toxic effects may be reversed by the administration of methionine. The effects may be produced in a variety of species, although there are differences in response. The rat also shows a sex difference in susceptibility, the female animal showing the toxic response rather than the male.

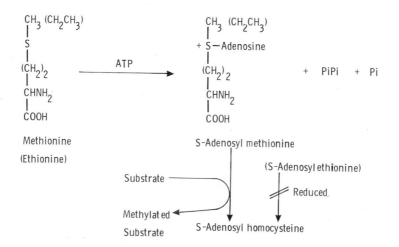

Figure 7.26. The role of methionine in methylation reactions and the mechanism underlying ethionine hepatotoxicity. After the substrate is methylated the *S*-adenosyl homocysteine remaining is broken down into homocysteine and adenine, both of which are re-utilized. When *S*-adenosyl ethionine is formed, however, this recycling is reduced (≠) and a shortage of adenine and hence ATP develops.

After a single dose of ethionine, triglycerides accumulate in the liver, the increase being detectable after four hours. After 24 hours the accumulation of triglycerides is maximal, being 15–20 times the normal level. Initially the fat droplets accumulate on the endoplasmic reticulum in periportal hepatocytes and then in more central areas of the liver. Some species develop hepatic necrosis as well as fatty liver, and nuclear changes and disruption of the endoplasmic reticulum may also be observed.

Chronic administration causes proliferation of bile duct cells leading to hepatocyte atrophy, fibrous tissue surrounding proliferated bile ducts and eventually cirrhosis and hepatocellular carcinoma.

The major biochemical changes observed are a striking depletion of ATP, impaired protein synthesis, defective incorporation of amino acids, and the appearance of RNA and proteins containing the ethyl rather than the methyl group. The plasma levels of triglycerides, cholesterol, lipoprotein and phospholipid are all decreased.

The mechanism underlying this toxicity is thought to involve a deficiency of ATP. Methionine acts as a methyl donor *in vivo*, in the form of *S*-adenosyl methionine, and ethionine forms the corresponding *S*-adenosyl ethionine. However, the latter analogue is relatively inert as far as recycling the adenosyl moiety is concerned, and this is effectively trapped as *S*-adenosyl ethionine (figure 7.26). The resulting lack of ATP leads to inhibition of protein synthesis and a deficiency in the production of the apolipoprotein complex responsible for transporting triglycerides out of the liver. Consequently, there is an accumulation of triglycerides.

The reduction in protein synthesis obviously has other ramifications, such as a deficiency in hepatic enzymes and a consequent general disruption of intermediary metabolism. Methylation reactions are presumably also affected.

S-Adenosyl ethionine carries out ethylation reactions or ethyl transfer and this is presumably involved in the carcinogenesis. Administration of ethionine to animals leads to the production of ethylated bases such as ethyl guanine. This may account for the observed inhibition of RNA polymerase and consequently of RNA synthesis. Incorporation of abnormal bases into nucleic acids and the production of impaired RNA may also lead to the inhibition of protein synthesis and misreading of the genetic code.

The depletion of ATP is the preliminary event leading to the pathological changes and the ultrastructural abnormalities of the nucleus and cytoplasmic organelles. Administration of ATP or precursors reverses all of these changes. The exact mechanism underlying the carcinogenesis is less clear, but presumably involves inhibition of RNA synthesis or the production of abnormal ethylated nucleic acids and hence disruption of transcription, translation or possibly replication. It is of interest that ethionine is not mutagenic in the Ames test, with or without rat liver homogenate. However, Weisburger (see Bibliography) has suggested that ethionine may be carcinogenic after metabolism to vinyl homocysteine (in which vinyl replaces ethyl) which is highly mutagenic.

Teratogenesis

Actinomycin D

Actinomycin D is a complex chemical compound produced by the *Streptomyces* species of fungus and is used as an antibiotic. It is a well established and potent teratogen and is also suspected of being carcinogenic.

The teratogenic potency of actinomycin D shows a marked dependence on the time of administration, being active on days 7–9 of gestation in the rat, when a high proportion of surviving foetuses show malformations (figure 6.10). Administration of the compound at earlier times, however (figure 7.27), results in a high foetal death and resorption rate. This falls to about 10% on the 13th day of gestation. The malformations produced in the rat are numerous, including cleft palate and lip, spina bifida, ecto and dextrocardia, anencephaly and disorganization of the optic nerve. Abnormalities of virtually every organ system may be seen at some time. Actinomycin D is

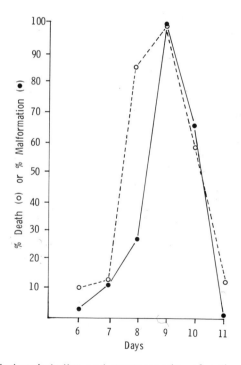

Figure 7.27. Embryolethality and teratogenecity of actinomycin D. This graph shows the relationship between the time of dosing and susceptibility to malformations (●) or death (○). Data from Wilson (1965) *Ann. N. Y. Acad. Sci.*, **123**, 119.

particularly embryolethal, unlike other teratogens such as thalidomide (see below). This embryolethality shows a striking parallel with the incidence of malformations (figure 7.28). Although this has been observed to a certain extent with some other teratogens, in other cases embryolethality and malformations seem to be independent variables. It is well established that actinomycin D inhibits DNA-directed RNA synthesis by binding to guanosyl residues in the DNA molecule. This disrupts the transcription of genetic information and thereby interferes with the production of essential proteins. DNA synthesis may also be inhibited, being reduced by 30–40% *in utero*. It is clear that in the initial stages of embryogenesis, synthesis of RNA for protein production is vital and it is not surprising that inhibition of this process may be lethal.

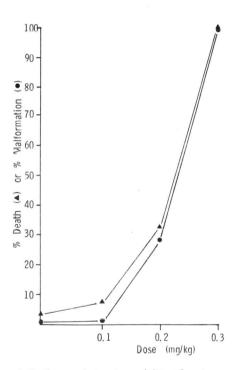

Figure 7.28. Embryolethality and teratogenicity of actinomycin D. This graph shows the dose–response relationship for these two toxic effects. Data from Wilson (1965) *Ann. N. Y. Acad. Sci.*, **123**, 119.

It has been shown that radiolabelled actinomycin D is bound to the RNA of embryos on days 9, 10 and 11 of gestation. Using incorporation of tritiated uridine as a marker for RNA synthesis, it was shown that only on gestational days 9 and 10 was there significant depression of incorporation in

I

certain embryonic cell groups. On days 7, 8 and 11 no significant depression of uridine incorporation was observed. The depression of RNA synthesis as measured by uridine incorporation therefore correlates approximately with teratogenicity. However, actinomycin D is also cytotoxic and this can be demonstrated as cell damage in embryos on days 8, 9 and 10 but not at earlier times or on day 11. Therefore, the teratogenesis shows a correlation with cytotoxicity as well as with inhibition of RNA synthesis. Certainly the concentration of actinomycin D in the embryo after administration on day 11 was too low for effective inhibition of RNA synthesis.

Although it is clear that actinomycin D is cytotoxic and inhibits RNA synthesis, the role of these effects in teratogenesis is not yet clear. RNA synthesis is a vital process in embryogenesis, preceding all differentiation, chemical and morphological, and therefore inhibition of it would be expected to disturb growth and differentiation. This may account for the production of malformations after administration on gestational day 7 in the rat, a period not normally sensitive in this species for the production of malformations. Excessive embryonic cell death may also be teratogenic.

Diphenylhydantoin

Diphenylhydantoin is an anticonvulsant drug in common use which is suspected of being teratogenic in humans. There is at present insufficient data available to specify the exact type of malformation caused in humans, but in a few cases craniofacial anomalies, growth retardation and mental deficiency have been documented. Heart defects and cleft palate have also been described in some cases in humans. In experimental animals, however, diphenylhydantoin is clearly teratogenic and this has been shown repeatedly in mice and rats. The defects most commonly seen are orofacial and skeletal, the orofacial defect usually described being cleft palate. Rhesus monkeys, however, are much more resistant to the teratogenicity, only showing minor urinary tract abnormalities, skeletal defects and occasional abortions after high doses.

Although the teratogenicity of diphenylhydantoin in humans has not been demonstrated so clearly as that of thalidomide, the levels of drug to which experimental animals were exposed were not excessively high. The plasma levels of the unbound drug in the maternal plasma of experimental animals after teratogenic doses were only 2–3 times higher than those found in man after therapeutic doses. The teratogenic effects in experimental animals were found to occur near the maternal toxic dose.

The types of defect produced in mice by diphenylhydantoin at various times of gestation are shown in table 7.5. There is good correlation between the timing of these defects and the known pattern of organogenesis in the mouse.

Table 7.5 Timing of teratogenic effect of diphenylhydantoin in the mouse.

Malformation	Treatment on gestational day					
	6–8	9–10	11–12	13–14	15–16	17–19
Orofacial	0	24	63	57	4	0
Eye defects	0	19	0	0	0	0
Limb defects	0	12	0	0	0	0
CNS defects	0	28	0	0	0	0
Skeletal defects	0	44	52	57	3	0
Kidney defects	0	25	17	7	4	0

Dose of diphenylhydantoin: 150 mg/kg.
Figures are percentages of all surviving foetuses displaying the malformation.
Data from Harbison, R. D. & Becker, B. A. (1969) *Teratology* **2**, 305.

It can be seen that the greatest number of malformations of any sort occur on gestational days 11–12, with these being mainly orofacial and skeletal.

Diphenylhydantoin induced malformations show a clear dose–response, as can be seen from figure 7.29 for pregnant mice treated on the 11th, 12th and 13th days of gestation. No significant increase in foetal deaths was observed below 75 mg/kg, but above this dose level more than 60% embryolethality was observed *in utero*, indicating a very steep dose–response curve. The mechanism underlying diphenylhydantoin teratogenicity is not fully understood, but enough is known to make it an interesting example.

In both rats and humans, diphenylhydantoin is known to undergo aromatic hydroxylation, presumably catalysed by the microsomal cytochrome P-450 system. However, pretreatment of pregnant mice with inducers or inhibitors of microsomal drug oxidation decreases or increases the teratogenicity respectively. This paradoxical effect may simply be due to increases or decreases in the removal of the drug from the maternal circulation by metabolism and excretion following pretreatment.

It has recently been proposed that metabolic activation of diphenylhydantoin may be responsible for the teratogenicity. After the administration of radioactively labelled diphenylhydantoin to pregnant mice, radioactive drug or a metabolite was found to be covalently bound to protein in the embryo. It was shown that both the teratogenicity and embryolethality of diphenylhydantoin could be increased by using an inhibitor of epoxide hydratase (see page 71), trichloropropene oxide. Similarly, the covalent binding of radiolabelled diphenylhydantoin to protein was also increased by this treatment.

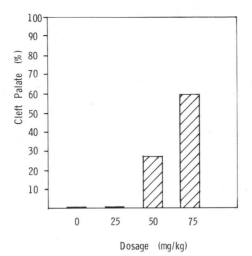

Figure 7.29. Dose–response relationship for diphenylhydantoin teratogenesis. The incidence of cleft palate in the surviving embryos is plotted against the dose of diphenylhydantoin given to pregnant mice on days 11, 12 and 13 of gestation. Adapted from Harbison & Becker (1969) *Teratology*, **2**, 305.

Metabolism by epoxide hydratase is effectively a detoxication pathway for reactive epoxides such as that proposed as an intermediate in diphenyl-hydantoin metabolism (figure 7.21), and inhibition of this enzyme therefore blocks the detoxication. It was postulated that the epoxide of diphenyl-hydantoin was the reactive and teratogenic intermediate produced by meta-bolism. The maternal plasma concentrations of drug in the mice used in this study were similar to those measured in humans after therapeutic doses of diphenylhydantoin had been given.

Although changes in the covalent binding of labelled diphenylhydantoin to foetal protein correlated with changes in teratogenicity, this does not prove a direct relationship. Whether the putative reactive intermediate of diphenyl-hydantoin which binds to protein is the ultimate teratogen awaits clarification.

Thalidomide

Despite the great interest in and notoriety of thalidomide as a teratogen, little information is available about the possible mechanism of its terato-genicity. It is, however, of particular interest in being a well established human teratogen.

Thalidomide was an effective sedative sometimes used by pregnant women for the relief of morning sickness, and the drug seemed remarkably non-toxic. However, it eventually became apparent that its use by pregnant women was associated with characteristic deformities in the offspring. These deformities were phocomelia (shortening of the limbs), and malformations of the face and internal organs have also occurred. It was the sudden appearance of cases of phocomelia which alerted the medical world, as this had been a hitherto rare congenital abnormality.

It became clear that in virtually every case of phocomelia, the mother of the malformed child had definitely taken thalidomide between the 3rd and 8th week of gestation. In some cases only a few doses had been taken during the critical period. Analysis of the epidemiological and clinical data suggested that thalidomide was almost invariably effective if taken on a few days or perhaps just one day between the 20th and 35th gestational days. It has been possible to pinpoint the critical periods for each abnormality. Lack of the external ear and paralysis of the cranial nerve occur on exposure during the 21st and 22nd days of gestation. Phocomelia, mainly of the arms, occurs after exposure on days 24–27 of gestation with the legs affected 1–2 days later. The sensitive period ends on days 34–36 with production of hypoplastic thumbs and anorectal stenosis.

Initially these malformations were not readily reproducible in rats or other experimental animals. It was later discovered that limb malformations could be produced in certain strains of white rabbits if they were exposed during the 8th–16th days of gestation. Several strains of monkeys were found to be susceptible and gave similar malformations to those seen in humans. It was eventually found that malformations could be produced in rats but only if they were exposed to the drug on the 12th day of gestation. At teratogenic doses thalidomide has no embryolethal effect, doses several times larger being necessary to cause foetal death.

The mechanism underlying thalidomide teratogenesis has never been completely elucidated, despite considerable research. However, the evidence suggests that a metabolite is responsible rather than the parent drug. The metabolism of thalidomide is complex, involving both enzymic and non-enzymic pathways. A number of metabolites arise by hydrolysis of the amide bond in the piperidine ring (figure 7.30) of which about 12 have been identified *in vivo*, and aromatic ring hydroxylation may also take place. The hydrolytic opening of the piperidine ring yields phthalyl derivatives of glutamine and glutamic acid. Phthalylglutamic acid may also be decarboxylated to the monocarboxylic acid derivative. Other monocarboxylic and dicarboxylic acid derivatives are also produced, some by opening of the phthalimide ring.

None of these metabolites was found to be teratogenic in the rabbit, but it has been subsequently found that they were unable to penetrate the embryo. Studies *in vivo* revealed that after the administration of the parent drug the major products detectable in the foetus were the monocarboxylic acid derivatives. It therefore seems that the parent drug may cross the placenta and enter the foetus and there be metabolized to the teratogenic metabolite.

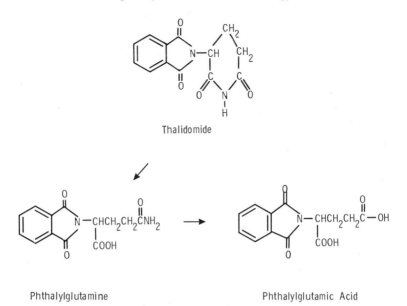

Thalidomide

Phthalylglutamine   Phthalylglutamic Acid

Figure 7.30. Structure of thalidomide and two of its hydrolysis products.

Subsequently the phthalylglutamic acid (figure 7.30), a dicarboxylic acid, was shown to be teratogenic in mice when given on days 7–9 of pregnancy. However, other work has indicated that the phthalimide ring is of importance in the teratogenicity. Other studies have indicated that thalidomide acylates aliphatic amines such as putrescine (figure 4.26) and spermidine, histones, RNA and DNA and that it may also affect ribosomal integrity. More recent work has suggested that a chemically reactive metabolite is the ultimate teratogen.

This metabolite is thought to be an epoxide. Hepatic microsomes from pregnant rabbits and hepatic preparations (S–9) from rabbit, monkey and human foetuses all produced a metabolite which was toxic to human lymphocytes *in vitro*. Liver microsomes from pregnant rats did not. This species difference is in agreement with the difference in susceptibility to thalidomide teratogenesis.

Furthermore, inhibition of epoxide hydratase increased and addition of the purified enzyme decreased the toxicity of thalidomide to human lymphocytes *in vitro*. This data suggested that an epoxide might be involved in the toxicity and this is supported by earlier metabolic studies *in vivo* which have shown the presence of phenolic metabolites in the urine of rabbits but not rats treated with the drug.

Perhaps the particular lesson to be learnt from the tragedy of thalidomide is that a drug with low maternal and adult toxicity, which is similarly of low toxicity in experimental animals, may have high teratogenic activity. The human embryo seems to have been particularly sensitive to normal therapeutic doses in this case. However, it has resulted in new drugs now being more rigorously tested and also tested in pregnant animals.

Immunogenesis

Practolol

Practolol (figure 7.31) is an antihypertensive drug which had to be withdrawn from general use because of severe adverse effects which became apparent in 1974 about four years after the drug had been marketed. The toxicity of practolol was unexpected and when it occurred it was severe. Furthermore, it has never been reproduced in experimental animals, even with the benefit of hindsight.

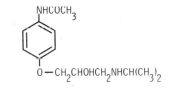

Figure 7.31. Structure of practolol.

The available evidence points to the involvement of an immunological mechanism, the basis of which is probably a metabolite–protein conjugate acting as an antigen. It seems unlikely that the pharmacological action of this drug, β-blockade, is involved, as other β-blocking drugs have not shown similar adverse effects. The syndrome produced by this drug features lesions to the eye, peritoneum and skin. Epidemiological studies have firmly established practolol as the causative agent in the development of this toxic effect, described as the occulomucocutaneous syndrome. This involved extensive and severe skin rashes, similar to psoriasis, and keratinization of the cornea and peritoneal membrane.

Studies *in vivo* showed that practolol was metabolized to a very limited extent in both human subjects and experimental animals. Furthermore, there were no antibodies demonstrable to practolol itself. However, in a hamster liver microsomal system *in vitro*, it was shown that practolol could be covalently bound to microsomal protein and also to added serum albumin. It was further shown that human sera from patients with the practolol syndrome contained antibodies which were specific for this practolol metabolite generated *in vitro*. Factors affecting the covalent binding of the practolol metabolite to protein *in vitro* also influenced the reaction between the patients' sera and the protein conjugate. The absence of NADPH, the presence of glutathione and the use of 3-methylcholanthrene-induced hamster liver microsomes, all reduced the binding and the immunological reaction. These results indicated a requirement for NADPH-dependent microsomal enzyme mediated metabolism and binding to protein to produce a hapten recognizable by the antibodies in the patients' sera.

The identity of the metabolite has not yet been established but it is neither the deacetylated nor 3-hydroxymetabolite found *in vivo*. However, deacetylation may be a prerequisite for the *N*-hydroxylation reaction which has been suggested.

Therefore it seems likely that practolol causes an adverse reaction which has an immunological basis due to the formation of an antigen between a practolol metabolite and a protein. The reason for the bizarre manifestations of the immunological reaction and the metabolite responsible have not yet been established.

Penicillin

Penicillin is a very widely used antibiotic drug, and is probably responsible for the majority of anaphylactic reactions. The incidence of allergic reactions to penicillin has been variously estimated as between 1 and 10% of recipients of the drug, but is probably in the region of 1–3%. The most common reactions are urticaria, skin eruptions and arthralgia. However, severe anaphylactic reactions (Type I, see page 161) may occur and can be life-threatening.

There may be several antigenic determinants for the one penicillin molecule, and these vary between individuals, so cross-reactivity may or may not occur with other penicillins. Also, IgM and IgG may act as blocking antibodies towards IgE, in which case anaphylactic reactions do not occur. This makes it difficult to predict the outcome of penicillin allergy.

The mechanism of penicillin immunotoxicity relies on the formation of a covalent conjugate with protein. This conjugate acts as an antigen. Penicillin undergoes slow transformation *in vivo* to a variety of products, some of which are chemically more reactive than the parent drug. The two derivatives of particular interest are penicillenic acid and penicilloic acid (figure 7.32). Penicillenic acid can react with the ε-amino group of lysine in proteins. The resulting α-amide derivatives of the penicilloic acid are thought to be the ultimate haptens (figure 7.32), and the penicilloic acid conjugate is the probable antigen in penicillin immunotoxicity. This was established in a number of studies using such techniques as hapten inhibition. This relies on the principle that the hapten or penicillin derivative combines with the antibody and therefore inhibits the antibody–antigen reaction (figure 6.14).

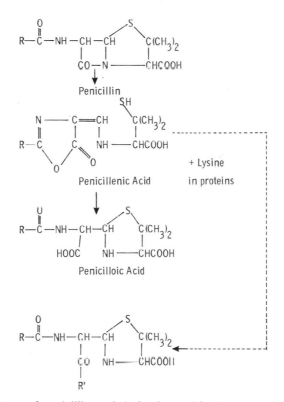

Figure 7.32. Structure of penicillin and derivatives arising by spontaneous transformation. For penicillin G, R = benzyl, R' = protein. Adapted from De Weck (1962) *Int. Archs Allergy appl. Immunol.*, **21**, 20.

This reaction is normally visualized as a precipitation or haemagglutination of the antibody–antigen complex.

Studies showed that the penicilloylamide conjugate with cysteine was a particularly strong inhibitor of the antibody–antigen reaction and was therefore a likely candidate for the hapten.

The case of penicillin allergy is probably one of the most understood, mechanistically, and supports the view that a drug–protein conjugate is the ultimate immunogen.

Hydralazine

Hydralazine is an antihypertensive drug which may cause a syndrome similar to the disease lupus erythematosus in 1–3% of recipients. This syndrome has features suggestive of an immunological type of toxicity such as the presence of antinuclear antibodies and antibodies to synthetic hydralazine–protein conjugates. The major manifestation of the syndrome is arthralgia.

Although the mechanism of hydralazine-induced lupus erythematosus has yet to be elucidated, certain aspects are of interest and illustrate the multifactorial nature of some drug toxicities. This syndrome has been found to occur more commonly in subjects with certain predisposing factors: it is more prevalent in women than in men by a factor of 4 : 1; it is very much more common in patients with the HLA type (tissue type) DR4; it occurs almost exclusively in patients with the slow acetylator phenotype; and it occurs more frequently after doses of more than 200 mg daily.

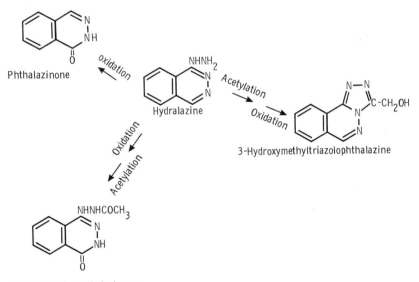

Figure 7.33. Some of the major routes of metabolism of hydralazine.

It has recently been shown that hydralazine metabolism is dependent on the acetylator phenotype in man, and it is postulated that oxidative routes of metabolism alternative to acetylation may produce the immunogenic metabolite (figure 7.33). These alternate routes of metabolism are clearly of more importance in the slow acetylator (figure 7.33). Although synthetic hydralazine–protein conjugates have been made and antibodies to them demonstrated, the structure of the conjugate, particularly that of the hydralazine moiety, is unknown.

This example of drug-induced immunotoxicity is important for two reasons.

(*a*) It illustrates the role of various factors in the production of toxicity, in this case an adverse drug reaction. The various factors mentioned mean that the expected occurrence of this adverse reaction would be in about 8% of recipients, if doses of 200 mg daily or greater were used. The doses currently used ensure that the incidence is in practice lower than 8%.

(*b*) It reveals the difficulties of testing for this type of reaction using experimental animals, when the various predisposing factors may not be present. For instance, the acetylator phenotype does not exist in most species of experimental animal and the immunological surveillance system and the HLA system are also different.

Metal toxicity

Mercury is an extremely toxic metal in its organic, inorganic and elemental forms. The mechanisms underlying its toxicity are partially understood and there are certain features in common with other metal toxicities, making it a good example to study.

Like certain other metals, mercury is a cumulative poison, accumulating because of the high affinity that tissues have for it. The metal is absorbed by most routes in the organic and salt forms, and the elemental vapour is absorbed by inhalation. Once mercury is absorbed and present in the plasma it can pass into the tissues, even crossing the blood–brain barrier in the organic and elemental forms.

Mercury in the organic form, such as methyl mercury, is particularly hazardous as, unlike elemental mercury, it is almost completely absorbed from the gastrointestinal tract, through the skin and via the lungs, and it has a longer biological half-life than the other forms. Mercury is often in this form in the environment, as it may be transformed to the organic form biologically. Methyl mercury was the infamous substance responsible for Minamata disease in Japanese people living around Minamata and ingesting mercury by eating fish from waters polluted with industrial effluent.

The half-life of mercury is relatively long: the initial phase, during which excretion is mainly foecal, is two days, and this is followed by a terminal phase with a half-life of about 20 days, when both foecal and urinary excretion occur. In rats, methyl mercury is excreted in the bile as a cysteine conjugate, is bound to protein and undergoes extensive enterohepatic circulation. Methyl mercury may also be biotransformed to inorganic mercury, which is excreted in the faeces.

Elemental mercury is oxidized *in vivo* to inorganic mercury, which is selectively accumulated in kidney tissue during excretion and also by the lysosomes.

The toxic effects of mercury are mainly damage to the central nervous system and to the kidney. Mercuric chloride causes severe kidney damage in both experimental animals and man. It seems that the proximal convoluted tubule is the prime target (see page 134). Methyl mercury is known to cause cerebral palsy and mental retardation in human children when they have been exposed *in utero*. This occurs after exposure of the mother during pregnancy to concentrations which have no apparent toxicity to the maternal system.

Mercury is a reactive element and its toxicity is probably due to its reactions with proteins. It binds to sulphydryl groups in proteins and is therefore an inhibitor of numerous enzymes, such as membrane ATPase. It may also react with amino, phosphoryl and carboxyl groups. Consequently, enzymes which are sulphydryl-dependent are inactivated by mercury, although this is usually reversible if the mercury is removed. Brain pyruvate metabolism is known to be inhibited by mercury, as are lactate dehydrogenase and fatty acid synthetase. The accumulation of mercury in lysosomes increases the activity of the lysosomal acid phosphatase. This may be a major cause of toxicity, as lysosomal damage releases various hydrolytic enzymes into the cell which then cause cellular damage.

Bibliography

General

BHATNAGAR, R. S. (1980) (editor) *Molecular Basis of Environmental Toxicity* (Ann Arbor: Ann Arbor Science Publications).

DOULL, J., KLAASSEN, C. D. & AMDUR, M. O. (1980) (editors) *Casarett and Doull's Toxicology, The Basic Science of Poisons* (New York: Macmillan).

GILLETTE, J. R. & MITCHELL J. R. (1975) Drug actions and interactions: Theoretical considerations. In *Handbook of Experimental Pharmacology*, Vol. 28, Part 3, *Concepts in Biochemical Pharmacology*, edited by J. R. Gillette and J. R. Mitchell (Berlin: Springer Verlag).

GILLETTE, J. R. & POHL, L. R. (1977) A prospective on covalent binding and toxicity. *J. Toxicol. Environ. Health*, **2**, 849.

GOLDSTEIN, A., ARONOW, L. & KALMAN, S. M. (1974) *Principles of Drug Action: The Basis of Pharmacology* (New York: John Wiley).

HODGSON, E. & GUTHRIE, F. E. (1980) (editors) *Introduction to Biochemical Toxicology* (New York: Elsevier-North Holland).

HODGSON, E., BEND, J. R. & PHILPOT, R. M. (1971–1981) *Reviews in Biochemical Toxicology*, Vols. 1–3 (New York: Elsevier-North Holland).

JOLLOW, D. J., KOCSIS, J. J., SNYDER, R. & VANIO, H. (editors) (1977) *Biological Reactive Intermediates* (New York: Plenum Press).

MITCHELL, J. R., POTTER, W. Z., HINSON, J. A., SNODGRASS, W. R., TIMBRELL, J. A. & GILLETTE, J. R. (1975) Toxic drug reactions. In *Handbook of Experimental Pharmacology*, Vol. 28, Part 3, *Concepts in Biochemical Pharmacology*, edited by J. R. Gillette and J. R. Mitchell (Berlin: Springer Verlag).

SLATER, T. F. (1972) *Free Radicals in Tissue Injury* (London: Pion).

SLATER, T. F. (editor) (1978) *Biochemical Mechanisms of Liver Injury* (London: Academic Press).

SMITH, D. A. (editor) (1977) Mechanisms of molecular and cellular toxicology. *J. Toxicol. Environ. Health*, **2**, 1229.

SNYDER, R., PARKE, D. V., KOCSIS, J., JOLLOW, D. J. & GIBSON, C. G. (editors) (1981) *Biological Reactive Intermediates 2: Chemical Mechanisms and Biological Effects* (New York: Plenum Press).

Symposium on Influence of Metabolic Activations and Inactivations on Toxic Effects. *Archs Toxicol.*, **39**, 1.

WITSCHI, H. & HASCHEK, W. M. (1980) Some problems correlating molecular mechanisms and cell damage. In *Molecular Basis of Environmental Toxicity*, edited by R. S. Bhatnagar (Ann Arbor: Ann Arbor Science Publications).

Chemical carcinogenesis

BROOKES, P. (1977) Role of covalent binding in carcinogenecity. In *Biological Reactive Intermediates*, edited by D. J. Jollow, J. J. Kocsis, R. Snyder and H. Vanio (New York: Plenum Press).

CLAYSON, D. B. & GARNER, R. C. (1976) Carcinogenic aromatic amines and related compounds. In *Chemical Carcinogens*, edited by C. E. Searle (Washington, D.C.: American Chemical Society).

DIPPLE, A. (1976) Polynuclear aromatic carcinogens. In *Chemical Carcinogens*, edited by C. E. Searle (Washington, D.C.: American Chemical Society).

HOLBROOK, D. J. (1980) Chemical carcinogenesis. In *Introduction to Biochemical Toxicology*, edited by E. Hodgson and F. E. Guthrie (New York: Elsevier-North Holland).

LAWLEY, P. D. (1980) DNA as a target of alkylating carcinogens. In *Chemical Carcinogenesis*, edited by P. Brookes, *British Medical Bulletin*, **36**, 19.

LEHR, R. E. & JERINA, D. M. (1977) Metabolic activation of polycyclic hydrocarbons. *Archs Toxicol.*, **39**, 1.

MAGEE, P. N. (1974) Activation and inactivation of chemical carcinogens in the mammal. In *Essays in Biochemistry*, edited by P. N. Campbell and F. Dickens, **10**, 105.

MAGEE, P. N., MONTESANO, R. & PREUSSMAN, R. (1976) *N*-Nitroso compounds and related carcinogens. In *Chemical Carcinogens*, edited by C. E. Searle (Washington, D.C.: American Chemical Society).

MILLER, E. C. & MILLER, J. A. (1976) The metabolism of chemical carcinogens to reactive electrophiles and their possible mechanism of action in carcinogenesis. In *Chemical Carcinogens*, edited by C. E. Searle (Washington, D. C.: American Chemical Society).

MILLER, J. A. & MILLER, E. C. (1977) The concept of reactive electrophilic metabolites in chemical carcinogenesis: Recent results with aromatic amines, safrole and aflatoxin B_1. In *Biological Reactive Intermediates*, edited by D. J. Jollow, J. J. Kocsis, R. Snyder and H. Vanio (New York: Plenum Press).

SIMS, P. (1980) Metabolic activation of chemical carcinogens. In *Chemical Carcinogenesis*, edited by P. Brookes, *British Medical Bulletin*, **36**, 11.

WEISBURGER, J. H. & WILLIAMS, G. M. (1980) Chemical Carcinogens. In *Casarett and Doull's Toxicology, The Basic Science of Poisons*, edited by J. Doull, C. D. Klaassen and M. O. Amdur (New York: Macmillan).

Tissue lesions

BOYD, M. R. (1980) Biochemical mechanisms in chemical induced lung injury: Roles of metabolic activation. *CRC Crit. Rev. Toxicol.*, **7**, 103.

GILLETTE, J. R. (1973) Factors that effect the covalent binding and toxicity of drugs. In *Pharmacology and the Future of Man, Proc. 5th Int. Congr. Pharmacology, San Francisco, 1972*, Vol. 2, edited by T. A. Loomis (Basel: Karger).

JOHNSON, M. K. (1975) The delayed neuropathy caused by some organophosphorus esters: mechanism and challenge. *CRC Crit. Rev. Toxicol.*, **3**, 289.

MAILMAN, R. B. (1980) Biochemical toxicology of the central nervous system. In *Introduction to Biochemical Toxicology*, edited by E. Hodgson and F. E. Guthrie (New York: Elsevier-North Holland).

MITCHELL, J. R., POTTER, W. Z., HINSON, J. A., SNODGRASS, W. R., TIMBRELL, J. A. & GILLETTE, J. R. (1975) Toxic drug reactions. In *Handbook of Experimental Pharmacology*, Vol. 28, Part 3, *Concepts in Biochemical Pharmacology*, edited by J. R. Gillette and J. R. Mitchell (Berlin: Springer Verlag).

RECKNAGEL, R. O. & GLENDE, E. A. (1973) Carbon tetrachloride hepatotoxicity: An example of lethal cleavage. *CRC Crit. Rev. Toxicol.*, **2**, 263.

RECKNAGEL, R. O., GLENDE, E. A. & HRUSZKEWYCZ, A. M. (1977) New data supporting an obligatory rule for lipid peroxidation in carbon tetrachloride-induced loss of aminopyrine demethylase, cytochrome P450 and glucose-6-phosphatase. In *Biological Reactive Intermediates*, edited by D. J. Jollow, J. J. Kocsis, R. Snyder and H. Vanio (New York: Plenum Press).

REYNOLDS, E. S. (1971) Liver endoplasmic reticulum: Target site of halocarbon metabolites. *Adv. exp. Med. Biol.*, **84**, 117.

SLATER, T. F. (1978) Biochemical studies on liver injury. In *Biochemical Mechanisms of Liver Injury*, edited by T. F. Slater (London: Academic Press).

TIMBRELL, J. A. (1979) The role of metabolism in the hepatotoxicity of isoniazid and iproniazid. *Drug. Metab. Rev.*, **10**, 125.

Exaggerated and unwanted pharmacological effects

GOLDSTEIN, A., ARONOW, L. & KALMAN, S. M. (1974) *Principles of Drug Action: The Basis of Pharmacology*, Chapter 5, Drug toxicity (New York: John Wiley).

MAIN, A. R. (1980) Cholinesterase inhibitors. In *Introduction to Biochemical Toxicology*, edited by E. Hodgson and F. E. Guthrie (New York: Elsevier-North Holland).

MURPHY, S. D. (1980) Pesticides. In *Casarett and Doull's Toxicology, The Basic Science of Poisons*, edited by J. Doull, C. D. Klaassen and M. O. Amdur (New York: Macmillan).

VESELL, E. S. (1975) Genetically determined variations in drug disposition and response in man. In *Handbook of Experimental Pharmacology*, Vol. 28, Part 3, *Concepts in Biochemical Pharmacology*, edited by J. R. Gillette and J. R. Mitchell (Berlin: Springer Verlag).

Lethal synthesis and incorporation

PETERS, R. A. (1963) *Biochemical Lesions and Lethal Synthesis* (Oxford: Pergamon Press).

SLATER, T. F. (1978) Biochemical studies in liver injury. In *Biochemical Mechanisms of Liver Injury*, edited by T. F. Slater (London: Academic Press).

ZIMMERMAN, H. J. (1976) Experimental hepatotoxicity. In *Handbook of Experimental Pharmacology*, Vol. 16, Part 5, *Experimental Production of Disease*, edited by O. Eichler (Berlin: Springer Verlag).

Teratogenesis

GORDON, G. B., SPIELBERG, S. P., BLAKE, D. A. & BALASUBRAMANIAN, V. (1981) Thalidomide teratogenesis: Evidence for a toxic arene oxide metabolite. *Proc. natn. Acad. Sci. USA*, **78**, 2545.

HARBISON, R. D. (1980) Teratogens. In *Casarett and Doull's Toxicology, The Basic Science of Poisons*, edited by J. Doull, C. D. Klaassen and M. O. Amdur (New York: Macmillan).

KEBERLE, H., LOUSTALOT, P., MALLER, P. K., FAIGLE, J. W. & SCHMID, K. (1965) Biochemical effects of drugs on the mammalian conceptus. *Ann. N.Y. Acad. Sci.*, **123**, 252.

LENZ, W. (1965) Epidemiology of congenital malformations. *Ann. N.Y. Acad. Sci.*, **123**, 228.

MARTZ, F., FAILINGER, C. & BLAKE, D. A. (1977) Phenytoin teratogenesis: correlation between embryopathic effect and covalent binding of a putative arene oxide metabolite in gestational tissue. *J. Pharmac. exp. Ther.*, **203**, 231.

WILLIAMS, R. T. (1963) Teratogenic effects of thalidomide and related substances. *Lancet*, **1**, 723.

WILSON, J. G. (1965) Embryological considerations in teratology. *Ann. N.Y. Acad. Sci.*, **123**, 219.

WILSON, J. G. & FRASER, F. C. (1977) *Handbook of Teratology*, Vol. 2 (New York: Plenum Press).

Immunogenesis

AMOS, H. E. (1979) Immunological aspects of practolol toxicity. *Int. J. Immuno-pharmac.*, **1**, 9.

GOLDSTEIN, A., ARONOW, L. & KALMAN, S. M. (1974) *Principles of Drug Action: The Basis of Pharmacology*, Chapter 7, Drug allergy (New York: John Wiley).

PERRY, H. M. (1973) Late toxicity to hydralazine resembling systemic lupus erythematosus or rheumatoid arthritis. *Am. J. Med.*, **54**, 58.

TIMBRELL, J. A., FACCHINI, V., STREETER, A. J., HARLAND, S. J. & MANSILLA-TINOCO, R. (1981) Lessons from other drug reactions: Hydralazine. In *Drug Reactions and the Liver*, edited by M. Davis, J. M. Tredger and R. Williams (Tunbridge Wells: Pitman Medical).

Metal toxicity

DONALDSON, W. E. (1980) Trace element toxicity. In *Introduction to Biochemical Toxicology*, edited by E. Hodgson and F. E. Guthrie (New York: Elsevier-North Holland).

HAMMOND, P. B. & BELILES, R. P. (1980) Metals. In *Casarett and Doull's Toxicology, The Basic Science of Poisons*, edited by J. Doull, C. D. Klaassen and M. O. Amdur (New York: Macmillan).

Glossary of Terms and Abbreviations

Å:	Angstrom unit; 1×10^{-8} cm
Acetyl CoA:	Acetyl coenzyme A
Acinus:	The functional unit of liver parenchyma
ADP:	Adenosine diphosphate
Allele:	One of two or more forms of a gene
Anaphylaxis:	An exaggerated allergic reaction to foreign substances
Androgens:	Male sex hormones
Anencephaly:	Congenital absence of the whole or part of the brain
Anoxia:	Deficiency of oxygen in the tissues
Antibody:	Specific protein produced in response to and to react with a foreign substance or body
Antigen:	A substance or structure capable of inducing the formation of antibodies
Apnea:	Cessation of breathing
Arthralgia:	Pain in a joint
Ataxia:	Failure of muscular co-ordination
ATP:	Adenosine triphosphate
ATPase:	Adenosine triphosphatase
Autosomal:	Relating to pairs of chromosomes other than the sex chromosomes
Bimodal distribution:	Having two modes or peaks
Bu:	Butyl, $CH_3CH_2CH_2CH_2$
Carcinogen:	Substance that induces cancer

233

Chromatids: Daughter strands of a duplicated chromosome joined by a centromere

Clara cell: Non-ciliated cell found in the terminal bronchioles of the lung

CNS: Central nervous system

CoA: Coenzyme A

Complement: Series of serum proteins concerned with reacting with the antigen-antibody complex

Crigler-Najjar Syndrome: Inherited metabolic disease which involves the absence of glucuronyl transferase giving rise to high levels of unconjugated bilirubin in the plasma

Cyt. P450: Cytochrome P450

Cytotoxic: Toxic to cells

Cytotropic antibodies: Antibodies having an affinity for cells

DDT: Dichlorodiphenyltrichloroethane

Dextrocardia: Location of the heart to the right of the thorax

Diploid: Having two sets of (homologous) chromosomes

Diuresis: Increased secretion of urine

DNA: Deoxyribonucleic acid. A polymer of deoxyribonucleotides forming the backbone of the chromosome and containing the genetic code

Down's Syndrome: Mongolism or Trisomy 21; due to presence of an extra chromosome

Dysarthria: Imperfect articulation of speech due to a disturbance of muscular control resulting from interference with the central or peripheral nervous system

Ectocardia: Congenital displacement of the heart

Ectoderm: Outermost of three primary germ layers of embryo

ED_{50}: Effective dose for 50% of the population

Endoderm:	Innermost of the three primary germ layers of the embryo
Enterohepatic circulation:	Circulation of a compound between the liver and gastrointestinal tract by excretion and reabsorption
Epidemiological:	Relation of the various factors determining the frequency and distribution of diseases
Epigenetic:	(In carcinogenesis) The induction of cancer without interaction with genetic material
Et:	Ethyl; CH_3CH_2
FAD:	Flavin adenine dinucleotide
Germ cells:	Gametes
Gilbert's Disease:	Inherited metabolic disease resulting in hyperbilirubinaemia
GSH:	Glutathione; γ-glutamyl-cysteinyl-glycine
Haemagglutination:	Agglutination of red blood cells
Haploid:	Having a single set of chromosomes as a result of meiotic division
Hapten:	Substance able to interact with an antibody when part of an antigen but not able to elicit the formation of an antibody alone
Heterozygous:	Possessing different alleles at a given locus
HLA:	Histocompatibility antigens on the surface of nucleated cells determined by a single major chromosomal locus, the HLA locus
Homozygous:	Possessing the same alleles at a given locus
Hyperbilirubinaemia:	High plasma bilirubin
Hypoglycaemia:	Low blood glucose
Hypoplastic:	Incompletely developed organ or structure
Hypotensive:	Low blood pressure

Ig:	Immunoglobulin; one of five classes: IgA, IgD, IgE, IgG or IgM
i.m.:	Intramuscular (injection)
in vitro:	In an artificial environment
in vivo:	In the living body
i.p.:	Intraperitoneal (injection)
i.r.:	Intrarectal (injection)
Ischaemia:	Deficiency of blood in a tissue
i.v.:	Intravenous (injection)
Keratinization:	Development of or conversion into keratin
K_m:	Michaelis-Menten constant. A parameter describing the affinity of an enzyme for its substrate. The substrate concentration at half maximal velocity
Kwashiorkor:	Disease in children produced by severe protein deficiency
LD_{50}:	Lethal dose for 50% of the population
Lupus Erythematosus (systemic):	Generalized connective tissue disorder characterized by autoimmune phenomena. Similar to rheumatoid arthritis
Lymphadenopathy:	Disease of the lymph nodes
3-MC:	3-Methylcholanthrene
Me:	Methyl; CH_3
Meiosis:	Cell division resulting in the production of haploid gametes
Mesoderm:	Middle layer of the three primary germ layers in the embryo
Methaemoglobinaemia:	Presence of oxidized haemoglobin or methaemoglobin in the blood
Microsomal:	The fraction of the cell homogenate in which particles of the smooth endoplasmic reticulum sediment
Mitosis:	Cell division resulting in the production of diploid daughter cells
NAD(H):	Nicotinamide adenine dinucleotide (reduced)

NADP(H):	Nicotinamide adenine dinucleotide phosphate (reduced)
Neonate:	New born animal
Neoplastic:	Pertaining to the abnormal growth of cells
Nystagmus:	Involuntary rapid movement of the eyeball
Oedema:	Presence of abnormally large amounts of fluid in the inter-cellular spaces
Ototoxicity:	Toxicity involving the eighth cranial nerve or the organs of hearing and balance
PAPS:	3-Phosphoadenosine-5-phospho-sulphate
Percutaneous:	Through the skin
Phagocytosis:	The engulfing of foreign particles by phagocytes
Phenotype:	The sum of the characteristics manifested by an organism as determined by genetics and environment
Phocomelia:	Developmental abnormality characterized by shortening of the limbs resulting from absence of the proximal section
Pinocytosis:	The uptake of liquids by cells involving the invagination of the cell membrane
pK_a:	Negative logarithm of the dissociation constant. The pH at which the compound is 50% ionized
p.o.:	Per os; oral (administration)
Polymorphism (genetic):	Two or more genetically determined phenotypes
Polyploidy:	Having more than two full sets of homologous chromosomes
Primordial:	Of the simplest and most undeveloped character
Probit (units):	Normal deviate of Gaussian curve plus 5

Psoriasis: Type of skin lesion or dermatosis

Radical: Molecular species having an unpaired electron

Replication: (Of DNA) Reproduction of an identical molecule

RNA: Ribonucleic acid. One of three forms, mRNA, messenger RNA, rRNA, ribosomal RNA or tRNA, transfer RNA

s.c.: Sub-cutaneous (injection)

SKF 525A: β-Diethylaminoethyl diphenyl-propylacetate; inhibitor of drug metabolism

S–9: The supernatant fraction of a cell homogenate following centrifugation at 9000 g for 10 minutes

Soluble fraction: Supernatant fraction of cell homogenate remaining after ultracentrifugation to remove organelles

Somatic cells: The cells of an organism other than the germ cells

Spina bifida: Developmental abnormality involving defective closure of the bony encasement of the spinal cord

SRSA: Slow reacting substance of anaphylaxis

TCA: Tricarboxylic acid cycle; Krebs cycle

TCDD: 2,3,7,8-Tetrachlorodibenzo-*p*-dioxin

TD_{50}: Toxic dose for 50% of the population

Transcription: Production of mRNA using DNA as a template

Translation: Process of information transfer from mRNA for protein synthesis

Trisomy 21: Downs Syndrome; presence of an additional chromosome

Tritiated:	Labelled with tritium, ^{3}H, a radioactive isotope of hydrogen
UDP:	Uridine diphosphate
UDPG:	Uridine diphosphate glucose
UDPGA:	Uridine diphosphate glucuronic acid
Urticaria:	Vascular reaction of the skin giving rise to weals and sometimes itching. Also known as hives
UTP:	Uridine triphosphate
Vasodilation:	Dilation of the blood vessels
Ventricular tachycardia:	Excessively rapid ventricular beat
V_{max}:	Maximum velocity of an enzyme reaction

Index

240